1

Aids to Physiotherapy

Aids to Physiotherapy

Edited by

Jennifer M. Lee
MSc BA MCSP DipTP

Principal Lecturer, Department of Health
and Community Studies, Teesside Polytechnic,
Middlesbrough

SECOND EDITION

CHURCHILL LIVINGSTONE
EDINBURGH LONDON MELBOURNE AND NEW YORK 1988

CHURCHILL LIVINGSTONE
Medical Division of Longman Group UK Limited

Distributed in the United States of America by
Churchill Livingstone Inc., 1560 Broadway, New
York, N.Y. 10036, and by associated companies,
branches and representatives throughout the
world.

First edition 1978
Second edition 1988

ISBN 0-443-03438-9

British Library Cataloguing in Publication Data
Aids to physiotherapy.
    1. Man. Diseases — For physiotherapy
    I. Lee, Jennifer M.
    616'.0024616

Library of Congress Cataloging in Publication Data
Aids to physiotherapy/edited by Jennifer M. Lee.
    — 2nd ed. p.   cm.
    Includes bibliographies and index.
    1. Physical therapy.   I. Lee, Jennifer M.
    [DNLM: 1. Physical Therapy — outlines.   WB
    18 A288]
    RM700.A66 1988   615.8   dc19   87-37853

Produced by Longman Singapore Publishers (Pte) Ltd.
Printed in Singapore.

Preface

The second edition of this book has undergone a major review in all sections; some sections have been rewritten – cardiorespiratory diseases, general surgery, diseases of the nervous system, fractures and orthopaedics, care of the elderly and paediatrics. A new section to cover the management of mental handicap has been included.

The book is primarily aimed at the senior student physiotherapist, although the newly qualified may also find it of help as well as those returning to practise after a break of two or three years. It is suggested that readers use this book as they would any set of 'notes' – to refresh the memory and 'cue' further thought processes. The book is designed as an *aide-mémoire*: it is not intended to be used in isolation but in association with books gleaned from the reading lists which can be found at the end of each section.

Middlesbrough, 1988   J.L.

Acknowledgements

I would like to thank all the contributors to the new edition of this book for their hard work and expertise in revising and rewriting the various sections. My thanks must also be extended to the staff of Churchill Livingstone, whose help I gratefully acknowledge. Finally, to the many unnamed patients who have added to the knowledge of all of the contributors to this book – our thanks.

Contributors

Deputy Principal, School of Physiotherapy, Lee...

Senior Physiotherapist, Doncaster Health Authority

J. Wise MCSP
District Physiotherapist, North Tees Health Authority

S. J. Adams MCSP
Senior Physiotherapist, Doncaster Health Authority

A. Bailey MCSP
Superintendent Physiotherapist, Doncaster Health Authority

M. A. Banks BA MCSP
Lecturer, Queen's College, Glasgow

F. H. E. Barlow MCSP DipTP
Senior Physiotherapist, South Tyneside Health Authority

S. P. Christie MCSP
Senior Physiotherapist, Norfolk and Norwich Hospital, Norwich

P. Cole MCSP
Senior Physiotherapist, South Tees Health Authority

G. Dean MCSP
Senior Physiotherapist, Doncaster Health Authority

M. G. W. Hall MCSP
Superintendent Physiotherapist, Doncaster Health Authority

D. A. Hill BSc MCSP DipTP
Head of Department, School of Health Sciences, University of Ulster

J. Johnstone MCSP
Senior Physiotherapist, Doncaster Health Authority

J. King MCSP
Senior Physiotherapist, Doncaster Health Authority

J. A. Lamb BA FCSP DipTP
Senior Teacher, Queen Elizabeth School of Physiotherapy, Birmingham

J. M. Lee MSc BA MCSP DipTP
Principal Lecturer, Department of Health and Community Studies, Teesside
Polytechnic, Middlesbrough

C. Perrin MCSP
Superintendent Physiotherapist, Doncaster Health Authority

C. Rushton MCSP
Superintendent Physiotherapist, Endeavour School, Middlesbrough

H. Standeven MCSP DipTP
Deputy Principal, School of Physiotherapy, Leeds

J. Wilkinson MCSP
Senior Physiotherapist, Doncaster Health Authority

J. Wise MCSP
District Physiotherapist, North Tees Health Authority

Contents

Contents

1. Movement

CLINICAL ASSESSMENT OF JOINT MOVEMENT

Classification of joints
1. *Fibrous*
    (i) Bony surfaces joined by fibrous tissue
    (ii) Little appreciable movement
    (iii) Types e.g. suture, gomphosis and syndesmosis
2. *Cartilaginous*
    (i) Bony surfaces joined by cartilage
    (ii) Limited movement
    (iii) Types e.g. synchondrosis and symphysis
3. *Synovial*
    (i) Bony surfaces not joined
    (ii) Bony surfaces covered with hyaline cartilage
    (iii) Joint cavity
    (iv) Articular capsule
    (v) Synovial membrane
    (vi) Synovial fluid
    (vii) Ligaments
    (viii) Variety of movements possible
    (ix) Types include ball and socket, condylar, plane, hinge, ellipsoid, saddle not pivot

Normal limiting factors to movement
1. Ligaments
2. Joint surfaces
3. Muscles
4. Connective tissue
5. Other parts of body

Reasons for limitation of movement
1. Destruction of intra-articular structures
2. Displacement of intra-articular body
3. Muscle disorder e.g. spasm, spasticity, weakness, flaccidity
4. Superficial scar tissue
5. Extra-articular and muscle adhesions

1

Measurement of joint movement
1. Goniometer
2. Tracings
3. Ruler/tape measure
4. Mathematical determination
5. X-rays/photographs

Recording methods
1. Numerical recording
2. Joint diagrams
3. Cumulative measurements plotted on graph
4. X-rays/photographs
5. Computer

Principles of assessment of joint movement
1. Patient's notes
2. Symptomatic enquiry
3. Position patient with joint uncovered
4. Fixation of adjacent joints
5. Observe joint for posture, swelling, redness, muscle appearance, scars, skin colour and texture
6. Palpate for joint temperature, type and amount swelling, tenderness, normal shape of joint
7. Check movement
   (i) Actively for ability to do voluntary movement, limitation of movement, pain, co-ordination, trick movements, muscle weakness or spasm, skin contractions
   (ii) Passively for ease of movement, limitation, muscle weakness/spasm, pain, crepitus
   (iii) Resisted movement for power through range and pain
8. Function
   (i) Lower limb joints check gait, stairs, turning
   (ii) Upper limb joints check hand function
   (iii) Trunk joints check transfers
9. Check general posture
10. Record findings
11. Reassess periodically e.g. fortnightly intervals

Mobilization of joint movement

Local relaxation
1. Contrast method
2. Reciprocal method
3. Pendular movement
4. Rhythmical passive movements
5. Neuromuscular facilitation e.g. hold-relax, contract-relax, Bobath
6. Massage
7. Hydrotherapy

Passive movement
1. Relaxed
2. Forced
3. Stretch single and multi-joint muscles
4. Mobilizations
5. Auto-assisted pulley circuits

Active assisted movement
1. Pendular exercises
2. Suspension
3. Hydrotherapy
4. Neuromuscular facilitation

Free active movement
1. Eccentric and concentric muscle work through full range
2. Use of lever length of limb
3. Variations in starting position
4. Speed
5. Duration of exercise

To support functional range
1. Splints – serial, 'lively', supporting, collars, corsets

Electrical techniques used to improve joint movement
1. Heat – IRR, paraffin wax, hot packs, microwave, SWD
2. Ultrasound
3. Pulsed SWD
4. Interferential
5. Faradism

CLINICAL ASSESSMENT OF MUSCLE FUNCTION

1. Isotonic – concentric, eccentric
2. Isometric/static
3. Isokinetic

Range of muscle work
1. Outer – full stretch to mid-point contraction
2. Inner – mid-point to full contraction
3. Middle – middle outer to middle inner range

Group action of muscles
1. Agonists/prime movers – produce required movement
2. Antagonists – controlled relaxation to allow movement
3. Synergists – assist action of agonists
4. Fixators – stabilize attachments of agonists, antagonists and synergists

Cause of muscle weakness
1. Intrinsic muscle disease
2. Lower motor neurone lesion
3. Lesions AHC
4. Lesions of upper motor neurone
5. Disordered proprioceptive input
6. Ischaemia
7. Disuse atrophy
8. Joint disease
9. Psychological

Measurement of muscle function
1. Oxford scale
   0 – Nil contraction
   1 – Flicker contraction
   2 – Contraction if gravity counterbalanced
   3 – Contraction against gravity only
   4 – Contraction against gravity and weight
   5 – Normal function
2. Manual Muscle Examination Record using good, poor, nil to assess contraction
3. 1. Repetition maximum
4. Tensiometer

Recording methods
1. Numerical
2. Cumulative muscle chart
3. Force–velocity curve

Principles of assessment of muscle function
1. Read patient's notes
2. Symptomatic enquiry
3. Patient positioned and adequately undressed
4. Observation and measurement of muscle bulk
5. Comparison with 'normal' side
6. Assess muscle function i.e. Oxford scale in all ranges/subjective assessment of endurance
7. Check for pain on contraction
8. Identify spasm/spasticity/rigidity/flaccidity
9. Assess functional use of affected limb/trunk
10. Record findings
11. Reassess at weekly intervals

Prevention of muscle atrophy
1. Isometric exercises – for painful/immobilized joints
2. Isotonic exercises – for pain free and mobile joints
3. PNF – facilitate contraction

4. Passive movements – maintain proprioceptive input to AHC and cortex
5. Electrical procedures – faradism to initiate contraction: IDC to maintain muscle properties

Re-education of muscle
1. Hypotonicity – flaccidity
2. Hypertonicity – spasticity, spasm, rigidity
3. Strengthening
4. Endurance
5. Co-ordination of muscle activity

1. Hypotonicity
   Techniques for facilitating muscle contraction:
   (i) Fast brushing
   (ii) Facilitatory icing
   (iii) Vibration
   (iv) Slapping
   } individually or in combination to appropriate dermatome/muscle belly/tendon
   (v) Use of visual/auditory stimuli
   (vi) PNF – successive induction
   (vii) Righting and equilibrium reactions
   (viii) Irradiation from movement of strong muscle groups
   (ix) Longitudinal compression
   (x) Longitudinal 'pounding'
   (xi) Other Rood techniques
2. Hypertonicity
   (i) To reduce spasticity
       Positioning:
       a. Bobath inhibitory position
       b. Shaking
       Movement:
       a. Reciprocal relaxation
       b. PNF techniques e.g. hold – relax, slow reversals
       Passive movements – rhythmical
       Ice pack (20–30 min)
       Immersion in cold water (10 min)
       Relaxation – general
       Massage – rhythmical, deep kneading
       Heat – variable in effect
   (ii) Spasm – primary aim is to reduce pain and thereby spasm by
       a. Application of heat e.g. hot pack, IRR, SWD, microwave, US
       b. Application of cold e.g. ice pack, immersion, ice cube massage
       c. Ethyl chloride spray
       d. TNS

        e. Relaxation techniques
        f. Passive movement
        g. Maitland mobilizations
        h. Hydrotherapy
        i. Active assisted exercises e.g. pendular
        j. Free active exercises
        k. PNF e.g. hold – relax/contract – relax, slow reversals
    (iii) Rigidity
        a. Passive movements 'pumping up'
        b. Trunk rotation – limb rotation
        c. Use righting responses to gain movement
        d. Transfers
        e. Free active movement – facilitation of movement
           patterns
3. Increase muscle power
    (i) Isometric exercises
    (ii) Isotonic exercises: type muscle work, speed, lever length
    (iii) Manual resistance
    (iv) PNF
    (v) Progressive resistance exercises
    (vi) Brief maximal exercises
    (vii) Use of body weight
    (viii) Springs/weights
    (ix) Malleable resistances
    (x) Underwater resistance
    (xi) Static machines e.g. rowing machine
4. Increase muscle endurance
    (i) Isotonic exercises
    (ii) Progressive resistance exercises
    (iii) Use of body weight
    (iv) Springs
    (v) Static bicycle/rowing machine/treadmill
    (vi) Endurance gym circuit
5. Co-ordination of muscle activity
    (i) Mat exercises – transfers and stabilization
    (ii) Lateral trunk/girdle movements
    (iii) Joint appproximation
    (iv) PNF to limbs e.g. holds in range, slow reversals
    (v) Progression of starting positions
    (vi) Balance and righting reflexes
    (vii) Weight-resisted exercises
    (viii) Frenkel's
    (ix) Functional activities

Co-ordination and balance

Control
1. Sensory input
   (i) Cutaneous
   (ii) Proprioceptive
   (iii) Special senses
2. Central co-ordination
   (i) Cerebrum and basal ganglia
   (ii) Brain stem nuclei
   (iii) Cerebellum
3. Effector system
   (i) Upper motor neurone pathways
   (ii) Lower motor neurone pathways

Causes of inco-ordination
1. Weak muscle groups
2. Pain/spasm
3. Spasticity
4. Loss of sensory input
5. Spinal cord lesion
6. Cerebellar lesion
7. Brain stem/basal ganglia lesion

Principles of treatment
1. Correct imbalance of muscle power
2. Relieve pain
3. Reduce spasticity
4. Inhibit formation or increase of spasticity

Use other intact senses to gain feed-back on body position.

Methods
1. PNF – rhythmic stabilizations, slow reversals
2. Approximation of joints
3. Progression of starting position
4. Balance and righting reflexes
5. Frenkels exercises
6. Functional activities

Re-education of gait

Assessment
1. Read patient's notes
2. Assess joint range and muscle power in lower limb
3. Analyse gait
4. Assess walking aid requirements
5. Assess muscle power in upper limbs

Preparation for walking
Aims to:
1. Strengthen extensor mechanism of upper limbs
2. Improve balance in sitting
3. Gain trunk mobility
4. Strengthen weight bearing limb
5. Teach hip hitching and active exercises to non-weight bearing limb
6. Ensure walking aid is correct size for patient
7. Demonstrate gait to patient
8. Teach sitting to standing and reverse
9. Teach gait

Methods of walking with aids
1. Non-weight bearing
2. Partial weight bearing
3. Full weight bearing

Types of aid
1. Crutches – axillary, elbow or gutter
2. Tripods/quadropods
3. Frame – fixed or reciprocal
4. Sticks

Aims of re-education of walking
1. To improve balance in standing
2. To teach turns, stairs, side-step and reverse steps
3. To progress gait pattern
4. To reduce support of aid
5. To analyse and correct gait faults

Some gait faults
1. Uneven step timing
2. Unequal length stride
3. Incorrect weight distribution on each foot
4. Abduction gait
5. Incorrect weight transference through weight bearing foot

Re-education of posture

Cause poor posture
1. Structural abnormalities
2. Muscle imbalance
3. Pain/tension
4. Neurological disorders
5. Debilitating disease
6. Occupational strains
7. Psychological

Assessment of posture
1. Patient's medical history
2. Observe static posture
   (i) From front, side, back
   (ii) Measure limb length
   (iii) Measure joint range
   (iv) Measure muscle strength
3. Observe dynamic posture
   (i) Trunk movements
   (ii) Feeding/dressing patterns
   (iii) Walking
4. Check for pain/spasm on movement
5. Test tendon reflexes
6. Record findings

Principles of treatment
1. Relieve pain
2. Gain relaxation of area
3. Mobilize affected joints
4. Strengthen weak muscles
5. Correct faulty muscle mechanics
6. Teach normal postural patterns by 'feel' and vision
7. Assess for supportive or corrective devices
8. Advice on home/occupational work postures

Methods
1. Heat e.g. IRR, SWD, microwave
2. Hydrotherapy/suspension
3. Active assisted/free active movements
4. Isometric exercises
5. Isotonic exercises
6. Manual, spring or weight resistance
7. Facilitation techniques
8. Balance boards
9. Teach back and neck care
10. Re-educate gait
11. Functional ADL activities

Re-education of respiratory movement

Cause of respiratory embarrassment
1. Respiratory and cardiac diseases
2. Structural disorders of thorax and vertebral column
3. Joint disease
4. Vascular disease
5. Postoperative lung infections

Assessment of respiratory movements
1. Read medical notes
2. Check posture and shape of chest
3. Assess chest expansion
4. Vitalograph readings
5. Cough and sputum
6. Range of movement in thoracic spine and shoulder girdle and joint
7. Exercise tolerance

See also pages 74 and 88.

Principles of treatment
1. Maintain clear airway
2. Teach correct breathing pattern
3. Remove secretions
4. Teach coughing
5. Improve movement in thorax, spine and shoulder girdle
6. Improve exercise tolerance

Methods
1. Relaxation general/local
2. Breathing exercises – general and local
3. Varying starting positions
4. Postural drainage
5. Cough-belt
6. Vibrations, shaking, percussion
7. General exercises, and posture correction
8. IPPB

See section on Cardiorespiratory disease page 71.

Hydrotherapy

Physiological effects
1. Rise in body temperature
2. Increased sweating
3. Superficial vasodilatation
4. Increase in peripheral circulation
5. Heart and respiratory rates increased
6. Blood pressure falls after immersion
7. Increased metabolism
8. Sedative effect on sensory nerve endings
9. Relaxation of muscle
10. Easily fatigued

Used to
1. Induce muscle relaxation
2. Relieve pain
3. Mobilize joints

4. Assist weak muscles to contract
5. Resist muscle work
6. Allows non-weight bearing walking
7. Encourage recreational activities
8. Achieve psychological effect

Disadvantages
1. Individual's fear of water
2. Rapid fatigue
3. Danger of infection
4. Difficult to fix joints and isolate movement

Procedure prior to entering pool
1. Read patient's notes
2. Check skin and continence
3. Assess mobility and strength
4. Explain treatment
5. Assess attitude to treatment
6. Patient takes shower
7. Enters antiseptic foot bath
8. Enters pool

Procedure after treatment
1. Shower
2. Pack in absorbent sheet and blanket
3. Bed rest for 20–30 min
4. Give drink
5. Dress
6. Allow further cooling off period prior to leaving building

Dosage
Start 5–30 min.

Contraindications
1. Skin infection or lesions
2. Cardiovascular disorders
3. Respiratory distress

Technical notes
1. Water temperature 34–37°C
2. Water changed every 4 h
3. Chlorination 0.5–0.75 parts per million
4. pH 7.2–8.0
5. Test pH and chlorination twice daily
6. Check stretchers, hoists and equipment weekly
7. Antiseptic foot bath changed twice daily
8. Pool area temperature 23–24°C
9. Changing area 18–19°C
10. Humidity 50–60%

Relaxation
Definition: muscles free from abnormal tension.

Causes of muscle tension
1. Disorders of CNS causing spasticity/rigidity
2. Pain causing spasm
3. State of mind

Methods of gaining relaxation of muscle
General relaxation:
1. Well-supported position
2. Quiet restful surroundings
3. Contrast method
4. Reciprocal method
Other techniques:
5. Hydrotherapy
6. Total suspension
7. Cold immersion techniques

Local relaxation
1. Contrast method
2. Reciprocal method
3. Yoga
4. Rhythmical passive movements
5. PNF e.g. hold – relax/contract – relax
6. Hydrotherapy
7. Local suspension
8. Free active pendular movements
9. Massage
10. Local heat e.g. hot packs, IRR, SWD, microwave
11. Local cold

2. Thermal, electrical and manipulative procedures

Physiological effects of local heat
1. Increased tissue metabolism, Van't Hoff's law
2. Increased superficial blood flow
3. Effect on sensory nerve endings
4. Relaxation of muscle tissue

More general effects
1. Fall in BP
2. Increase in heart and respiratory rate
3. Rise in 'core' temperature
4. Increased activity of sweat glands

Precautions for all heat treatments
1. Test integrity of skin thermal sensation
2. Check adequate circulation
3. Test understanding of patient
4. Read medical history
5. Warn patient re treatment

Dangers to use
1. Burns
2. Scalds
3. Syncope
4. Earth shock

SHORT WAVE DIATHERMY (SWD)

Technical notes
1. SWD uses wavelengths of the electromagnetic spectrum
2. Frequency 27 Hz
3. Wavelength 11 m
4. Depth of penetration – full body
5. Greatest heating in fat tissue
6. Heat produced in tissues by dipole rotation and molecular distortion/eddy currents
7. Applied using condenser field or cable technique

8. Condenser field produces electrostatic field
9. Cable produces electrostatic and magnetic field
10. Dosage
    Chronic conditions:
    (i) Intensity, comfortable-warmth
    (ii) Duration, maximum rise in tissue temperature at 20 min
    (iii) Frequency, daily
    Acute conditions:
    (i) Intensity, below sensation warmth
    (ii) Duration, $2\frac{1}{2}$–10 min
    (iii) Frequency, BD

Used to
1. Assist resolution of acute inflammation
2. Relieve pain
3. Increase vascularity
4. Induce muscle relaxation
5. Reduce viscosity of joint fluids and tissues

Contraindications
1. Large area loss of skin sensation
2. Venous thrombus
3. Arterial insufficiency
4. Haemorrhage
5. Metal in tissues
6. Pregnancy
7. Neoplasm
8. TB
9. Deep X-ray therapy
10. Cardiac pacemakers
11. Some intra-uterine devices

PULSED SHORT WAVE DIATHERMY

Technical notes
1. Pulsed SWD uses wavelengths of the electromagnetic spectrum
2. Frequency 27.12 MHz
3. Output 27–90 mW cm^2
4. Pulse length 65 s, resting pulse length 1600 s
5. Depth of penetration full body
6. Applied using condenser electrodes
7. Dosage 30 min
8. Produces pulsed electrostatic field

Used to
1. Assist resolution of inflammation
2. Relieve pain

3. Increase vascularity and reduce oedema
4. Enhance healing of tissues

Contraindications
As in SWD omitting (1), (9) and (10).

MICROWAVE

Technical notes
1. Microwave uses wavelengths of the electromagnetic spectrum
2. Frequency 2450 MHz wavelength 12.25 cm
3. Depth of penetration – 3 cm
4. Irradiates one surface of body
5. Greatest heating in vascular tissues cf. SWD
6. Heat produced in tissues by absorption of radiation and conduction in tissues
7. Eye protection for all treatments
8. Dosage up to 200 watts; 10–30 min, daily

Used to
1. Increase circulation
2. Raise threshold pain nerve endings
3. Reduce muscle spasm

Contraindications
1. Large area loss of thermal sensation
2. Not used near eyes, gonads, growing bone
3. Haemorrhage
4. Neoplasm and TB
5. Ischaemic conditions
6. Metal implants
7. Pregnancy
8. Severe oedema
9. Wet dressings

INFRA-RED RADIATION (IRR)

Technical notes
1. Non-luminous generator
2. Electromagnetic wavelength 4000–7700 Å
3. Shorter wavelengths produce greatest heating effect
4. Depth of penetration 1–10 mm
5. Heat produced by absorption of radiant energy
6. Dosage 20–30 min, daily
7. IRR obey optical laws

Used to
1. Relieve pain

2. Relax superficial muscle spasm
3. Increase superficial blood supply

Contraindications
1. Loss of large area of thermal skin sensation
2. Some skin diseases
3. Vascular insufficiency
4. Haemorrhage
5. Some skin liniments

ULTRASOUND (US)

Physiological effects
1. Thermal (unpulsed US)
   (i) Rise in tissue temperature, greatest in muscle
   (ii) Vasodilatation
2. Non-thermal (pulsed US)
   (i) Micromassage
   (ii) Analgesia

Technical notes
1. US is a form of acoustic vibration
2. Frequency 0.8–1 MHz, wavelength 1.5 mm
3. Depth of penetration varies with frequency and nature of tissue
4. Half value distance e.g. 1 000 000 Hz, $\frac{1}{2}$ value at 5 cm
5. Pulsed beam produces mechanical effect
6. Unpulsed beam produces thermal and mechanical effects
7. Dosage – acute conditions – 0.25–1.0 W/cm^2 BD 3 min
              chronic conditions – 1.0–3.0 W/cm^2 alt. days 8–10 min
   Depends on depth structure $\frac{1}{2}$ value distance
8. Application, either contact or immersion
9. Coupling medium usually necessary with stationary/moving head technique

Used to
1. Remove oedema
2. Increase blood supply
3. Reduce pain
4. Mobilize collagen tissues
5. Assist relaxation of muscle spasm

Contraindications
1. Care when treating areas adjacent to eyes, ear, testes and ovaries
2. Impaired circulation
3. Thrombus formation
4. Neoplasm and TB

5. Acute sepsis
6. DXRT and isotope treatment
7. Haemophiliacs

ULTRAVIOLET RADIATION

Physiological effects
1. Four degrees erythema reaction (2500 Å and 3000 Å)
2. Epidermal thickening
3. Desquamation
4. Pigmentation (2300–3400 Å)
5. Abiotic effect (2500–2700 Å)
6. Formation vitamin D (2800 Å)
7. Psychological effect

Technical notes
UVR part of:
1. Electromagnetic spectrum 3900–1849 Å
2. Depth of penetration 1.5 mm
3. Application in contact, 18 in or 36 in
4. Filters to absorb different wavelengths
5. Dosage
   skin test or E_1^0; to repeat E_1^0 add 25% previous dose
   E_2^0 is $E_1^0 \times 2\frac{1}{2}$; to repeat E_2^0 add 50% previous dose
   E_3^0 is $E_1^0 \times 5$; to repeat E_3^0 add 75% previous dose
   E_4^0 is $E_1^0 \times 10$; to repeat E_4^0 add 100% previous dose
   suberythemal dose $\frac{1}{2}$–$\frac{2}{3}$ of E_1^0
   To calculate dose at new distance:

   $$\text{New dose} = \frac{\text{Old dose} \times \text{new distance}^2}{\text{old distance}^2}$$

Used to
1. Stimulate growth of new skin
2. Produce pigmentation
3. Exfoliation
4. Improve superficial circulation
5. Heal wounds
6. Counter-irritant effect
7. Produce vitamin D
8. Reduce infection
9. Psychological effect

Contraindications
1. Individual sensitivity
2. Sensitizing drugs e.g. some antibiotics, tranquillizers, steroids
3. Certain diseases e.g. TB, eczema
4. Deep X-ray therapy

LOW FREQUENCY MUSCLE STIMULATING CURRENTS

Faradic type current

Physiological effects
1. Stimulation of sensory and motor nerve
2. Facilitate muscle contraction
3. Increase muscle metabolism
4. Vasodilatation of deep and superficial blood vessels
5. Increased arterial supply
6. 'Muscle-pump' action improves venous and lymphatic drainage

Used to
1. Re-education of muscle action
2. Train new muscle function
3. Increase circulation
4. Prevent/stretch adhesions
5. Hypertrophy muscle

Technical notes
1. Faradic type current is an alternating current
2. Pulse lengths 0.1–1.0 ms
3. Frequency 50–100 Hz
4. Surged
5. Dosage, cease when voluntary contraction achieved

Interrupted direct current

Physiological effects
1. Stimulation of sensory nerves
2. Contracts denervated muscle
3. Increases blood supply
4. Improves venous and lymphatic drainage
5. Chemical effects

Used to
1. Maintain properties of muscle
2. Improve circulation
3. Test muscle for re-innervation (SDC)
4. Prevent contractures

Technical notes
1. Depolarized IDC
2. Pulse length between 300 ms–0.03 ms
3. Pulse shape: triangular, trapezoidal, saw tooth square wave
4. Frequency 30 impulses per min, can be varied
5. Dosage: minimum of 90 contractions per muscle per day

Interferential

Allows low frequency stimulation without the problem of high skin resistance.

2 low frequency circuits 1 at 4000 Hz the other at 3900–4000 Hz.

The 2 circuits 'interfere' with each other and have a beat frequency of 0–100 Hz, used with 4 electrodes (2 for each circuit). Selection of frequencies determines the effect:

1. 0–10 Hz stimulates innervated muscle
2. 0–100 promotes blood and lymphatic circulation
3. 90–100 induces pain relief and relaxation

Contraindications to use
1. Arterial disease
2. Thrombus formation
3. Any acute infection

TRANSCUTANEOUS ELECTRICAL NERVE STIMULATION (TNS)

1 output 0–50 mA, frequency 15–200 Hz, pulse width 0.1–0.5 ms. 2 types high and low frequency TNS, applied via surface electrodes.

1. High frequency, low intensity TNS
2. 10–100 Hz, low current intensity for approx. 30 min
3. Effects – evokes 'pain gate' theory mechanism to relieve pain
4. Application – over peripheral nerve trunk or over a superficial cutaneous branch supplying painful area
5. Low frequency high intensity TNS
6. 50–100 Hz frequency in a train of 1–5 Hz stimuli, for > 30 min
7. Effects – stimulates the release of endorphins and endogenous opiates
8. Application – place cathode distal to the pain and anode over site of pain, or electrodes are diagonally placed around painful area

BIOFEEDBACK

The recording of physiological activity in the body which is presented as visual and/or auditory stimuli.

Either ECG or EMG feedback is used (electrocardiogram and electromylogram respectively):

1. ECG subject tries to reduce heart rate by concious effort
2. EMG subject tries to reduce frequency and size of 'spike' potentials or to reduce auditory stimuli

Uses
1. ECG for relaxation
2. EMG
     (i) To regain normal tone in hypo or hypertonicity
     (ii) For relaxation in relief of pain and posture re-education

  (iii) Re-education of gait and balance reactions
  (iv) To retrain weight transference in different starting
        positions
   (v) To re-educate awareness of body image

COLD THERAPY

Physiological effects of local cold

Effect on nerve tissue
1. Brief cutaneous cooling 3–5 s increases input to CNS and
   enhances motor output
2. Longer period of cooling 5–7 min diminishes sensation
3. Prolonged period of cooling 20–30 min diminishes muscle tone
   and nerve conduction velocity

Effect on circulation
1. Vasoconstriction initially on application
2. Vasodilatation later in cold application

Effect on tissues
1. Reduces metabolic rate
2. Increases joint viscosity
3. Increases muscle viscosity
4. Produces longer contraction and relaxation time in muscle

Precautions
1. Care in arteriosclerotic heart disease
2. Ischaemic tissue
3. Hypertension – with care
4. Psychological
5. No cold to cutaneous area of vagus nerve

Contraindications
1. Circulatory disorders
2. Coronary heart disease
3. External haemorrhage
4. Cold allergy
5. Cold aversion

Used to
1. Control oedema formation and haemorrhage
2. Relieve pain
3. Reduce muscle spasm
4. Reduce muscle spasticity
5. Improve nerve transmission
6. Increase visual acuity
7. Facilitate muscle contraction
8. Improve sustained muscle contraction

Methods of application
1. Cold pack
2. Cold immersion of limb or lower trunk
3. Ice cube massage
4. Ethyl chloride spray
5. Contrast baths

MANIPULATIVE PROCEDURES

Terminology

Effleurage	– stroking, gliding movements
Petrissage	– compression movements
Friction	– deep local massage
Vibration	– oscillatory to-and-fro movements
Percussion	– clapping
Tapotement	– percussion

EFFLEURAGE

Effleurage
1. Rhythmical
2. Deep/superficial centripetal gliding movements
3. One or two handed

Effects
1. Increases superficial lymphatic and venous flow
2. Mobilization of superficial soft tissues
3. Stimulates 'axon reflex'

Used to
1. Remove oedema
2. Stretch scar tissue
3. Relax muscles

Stroking
1. Rhythmical, superficial/deep movements
2. Speed variable
3. One or two handed

Effects
1. Sedative or stimulating to nervous system
2. Brisk stroking produces superficial vasodilatation

Used to
1. Relieve local muscle spasm
2. General relaxation
3. Stimulate superficial vasodilatation

PETRISSAGE

Kneading
1. Using palm/finger(s)
2. Depth and speed variable
3. One or two handed

Picking up
1. Lifting and squeezing muscle
2. One or two handed

Wringing
1. Lifting, squeezing, wringing action of superficial soft tissues
2. Two handed

Skin rolling
1. Skin and subcutaneous tissues grasped and rolled between fingers
2. Two handed

Effects
1. Increase venous and lymphatic return
2. Superficial vasodilitation
3. Reduce muscle tone
4. Mobilize skin and fibrous tissue

Used to
1. Increase circulation
2. Sedative effect
3. Reduce spasm/spasticity
4. Mobilize scar tissue and adhesions

FRICTIONS
1. Circular/transverse movements
2. Using fingers of one or two hands
3. Pressure increase with application

Effects
1. Mobilize deep structures
2. Increases blood supply
3. Produces temporary analgesia
4. Reduces haematoma formation

Used to
1. Mobilize ligaments, tendons or tendon sheaths
2. Reduce haematoma

VIBRATION

Shaking
1. Rhythmic large amplitude shaking movement
2. One or two handed

Vibration
1. Rhythmic small amplitude movement
2. Constant manual pressure
3. One or two handed

Effects
To produce movement of gases and liquids

Used to
1. Remove secretions in lung
2. Reduce tissue effusion

TAPOTEMENT

Clapping
1. Relaxed, cupped hand
2. Alternate movement of hands

Effects
1. Mobilize secretions
2. Produces skin erythema

Used to
1. Remove bronchial secretions
2. Induce coughing
N.b. can increase pleural effusion.

JOINT MOBILIZATIONS

It is not intended to give details of mobilization techniques but to remind the student that these techniques are an important part of patient management and to refer the reader to other texts (see reading list).
Joint mobilizations include:
1. Relaxed passive joint movements
2. Joint mobilizations
    (i) Grade I: small amplitude movements at beginning of range of movement
   (ii) Grade 2: larger amplitude movements within range of movement
  (iii) Grade 3: large amplitude movements up to limit of range of movement

(iv) Grade 4: small amplitude movements at limit of range of
       movement

All mobilization grades of movement are performed either gently
or strongly with a moderate speed of amplitude.

The movements are under the control of the patient at all times.

Used to
1. Reduce pain
2. Improve range
3. Thereby restoring function

FURTHER READING

Coate, H. & King A. (1985) *Patient Assessment*. Edinburgh: Churchill
    Livingstone.

Duffield, M. H. ed. (1976) *Exercises in Water*. London: Bailliere.

Forster, A. & Palastanga, N. (1986) *Clayton's Electrotherapy and
    Actinotherapy*. 9th edition. London: Bailliere Tindall.

Gardiner, M. D. (1981) *Principles of Exercise Therapy*. London: Bell &
    Hyman.

Hollis, M. (1976) *Practical Exercise Therapy*. Oxford: Blackwell.

Lee, J. M. & Warren, M. P. (1978) *Cold Therapy in Rehabilitation*. London:
    Bell & Hyman.

Licht, D. ed. (1960) *Massage Manipulation and Traction*. New Haven: Licht.

Licht, S. ed. (1963) *Medical Hydrology*. New Haven: Licht.

Licht, S. ed. (1965) *Therapeutic Exercises*. New Haven: Licht.

Licht, S. ed. (1967) *Therapeutic Electricity and UltraViolet Radiation*. New
    Haven: Licht.

Maitland, G. D. (1981) *Peripheral Manipulation*. London: Butterworth.

Maitland, G. D. (1986) *Vertebral Manipulation*. London: Butterworth.

O' Connell A. L. & Gardner, E. B. (1972) *Understanding the Scientific Bases
    of Human Movement*. Baltimore: Williams and Wilkins.

Stillwell, K. (1983) *Therapeutic Electricity and Ultraviolet Radiation*.
    Baltimore: Williams & Wilkins.

Summer, W. & Patrick, M. K. (1964) *Ultrasonic Therapy*. Amsterdam:
    Elsevier.

3. Behavioural sciences

Behavioural science is the scientific study of behaviour and experience. Behaviour can be objectively observed and recorded. Experience is personal and subjective.

SCOPE OF BEHAVIOURAL SCIENCE

Considerable overlap exists between the following areas:
1. Developmental psychology
2. Comparative psychology
3. Physiological psychology
4. Educational psychology
5. Organizational psychology
6. Clinical psychology
7. Social psychology
8. Sociology

Different schools of psychology may appear to be contradictory, but are better regarded as complementary.

Behaviourists claim to be interested only in behaviour.

Cognitive schools study conscious awareness.

DEVELOPMENTAL PSYCHOLOGY

Aspects
1. Physical development and growth (dealt with in Anatomy and Physiology)
2. Mental and perceptual development
3. Moral development

Stages of mental and perceptual development (Piaget)

1. Sensory motor stage, birth – 18 months
Child is born with certain reflexes e.g. sucking, grasping. These reflexes are rapidly adapted into more purposeful movements in response to specific stimuli. There is little evidence of imagery, or mental representation of objects in the outside world.

2. Pre-operational stage, 18 months – 7 years
Simple rules of arithmetic can be learned, but their implications are not fully mentally internalized. The child is therefore unable to appreciate conservation of physical properties of volume, mass or number. Perceptions are always from child's point of view i.e. egocentric.

3. Concrete operational stage, 7–11 years
Child now appreciates conservation of volume, mass and number. Perception shows awareness of relationships between separate objects and concepts.

4. Formal operational stage, 11 years onwards
Child is able to appreciate abstract concepts concerning behaviour of objects in the physical world e.g. buoyancy, momentum, velocity. Also able to appreciate and formulate universal rules and scientific laws involved with such concepts.

Moral development
Up to the age of 6 years children tend to judge good behaviour as that which is rewarded, and bad behaviour as that which is punished. Judgement is based on the consequences of the bahaviour. By the age of 10 intentionality plays a more important role in judging moral behaviour. During adolescence strong attitudes concerning clusters of political or religious values may develop, but their intensity usually mellows with age.

Learning
A change in behaviour as the result of experience.

Types of learning

	Imprinting
Associative learning	Classical conditioning Operant conditioning Avoidance conditioning Habituation learning
	Latent learning
Cognitive learning	Imitation Insight Creativity

Imprinting
The tendency of the newborn to follow the first moving object it sees, which in natural conditions is the mother. It occurs particularly in species which are mobile from birth e.g. chickens, cattle. There is some doubt as to whether it occurs in humans.

Classical conditioning
Occurs when the autonomic nervous system responds to a previously neutral stimulus. The stimulus has to be associated with another stimulus to which the autonomic system already responds. For example, pain causes specific responses.

If the therapist causes pain, then the sight or thought of the therapist may be sufficient to evoke the autonomic responses to pain. Some attitudes are formed as a result of classical conditioning.

Operant conditioning
Occurs when the voluntary muscles are used in order to obtain a reward. The reward reinforces the behaviour, and makes its repetition more likely. For example, if a patient feels better after attending for treatment, he is more likely to attend in future.

Avoidance conditioning
Occurs when an individual learns to behave in such a manner that he avoids unpleasant stimuli. Punishment may be used as an avoidance conditioner, and may take various forms e.g. physical, verbal.

Using bio-feedback techniques, operant conditioning of the autonomic nervous system is now possible. Some medical implications are:
1. Voluntary regulation of blood pressure
2. Voluntary regulation of local body temperature (useful for migraine patients)
3. Voluntary regulation of EEG waves, which may be used to abort epileptic attacks

Habituation learning
A decreased response to repetitions of the same stimulus e.g. patient's anxiety responses may reduce with repeated visits for treatment.

Latent learning
Occurs in the apparent absence of either pleasant or unpleasant stimuli. Only neutral stimuli are present. Latent learning possibly satisfies a curiosity drive. Latent learning may prove useful at a later date.

Imitation learning
When the learner observes another's behaviour, and then matches their own behaviour to that of the observed model. This is formally used in demonstrations to students, patients etc.

Insight learning
Problem solving. The individual draws on past experience to arrive at a solution which often occurs in 'a flash of inspiration'.

Creativity
The production of a completely new set of ideas. Inventiveness, or
originality of thought in art, science, music etc.

Motor skill
The learned ability to bring about predetermined results with
maximum certainty, often with the minimum outlay of time or
energy or both (Guthrie).
Most physiotherapy treatments involve the teaching of motor skills
to patients. Maturational skills e.g. walking rely on correct
neurological development.

Reasons for practice of a skill
1. To acquire a new skill
2. To improve an existing skill
3. To maintain a high level of skill

Guidance of a skill can
1. Reduce the errors during practice
2. Shorten the time necessary to acquire skill
3. Result in a higher ultimate level of skill

Types of guidance
1. Verbal (explanation)
2. Visual (demonstration)
3. Manual (assisted or resisted)
4. Mechanical (assisted or resisted)
   All types of guidance are relevant to physiotherapists especially
during muscle training or re-education.

Massed or spaced practice
In massed practice the skill is practised frequently with only short
intervals between practice sessions. In spaced practice the intervals
between sessions are longer.
   Optimum spacing varies with the complexity of the skill and the
personality of the learner. Complex skills benefit from greater
spacing.

Whole or part practice
The size or complexity of a skill will affect the optimum size of any
part of the skill which can be learnt at one practice session e.g. the
skill of manipulative treatments could not all be taught at one time.
Optimum size of part will also be affected by the capacity of the
learner, and should be considered for each patient learning or relearning a skill.

Knowledge of results (feedback)
The learner acquires skill more rapidly if he is well informed

concerning progress e.g. verbal reinforcement.

'Transfer' occurs when the learning of one skill affects the learning of another skill. Positive transfer facilitates learning between skills, and should be encouraged. Positive transfer occurs when the learning situation and skill requirements are similar e.g. practising walking on a smooth gymnasium floor may not show much positive transfer if the patient has to walk across a ploughed field to get home.

Intelligence

The level of adaptability to environmental requirements.

Measurement

Intelligence Quotient (IQ) is an attempt to assign a numerical value to intelligent behaviour, based on comparing mental age with chronological age, up to the age of 16.

$$IQ = \frac{Mental\ age}{Chronological\ age} \times \frac{1}{100}$$

The concept of IQ is carried on into adult life.

For any individual, intelligence levels tend to be general across wide areas of intellectual ability, but some variation does exist in different aspects of intelligence. Some people may score high on verbal and educational factors, while others may score high on mechanical and mathematical factors.

Evidence suggests that intelligence is mainly heredity, but can be influenced by extremes of environment.

Perception

The organism's interpretation of internal and external environmental stimuli.

Some perceptual abilities are either innate, or rapidly learned by the newborn infant e.g. perception of a human face.

Other perceptual abilities are greatly modified by environment and experience, especially during development e.g. perception of distances or angles.

Perceptual constancy

People tend to perceive what they expect to perceive e.g. oval coins tend to be perceived as round. Pictures of grass tend to be perceived as green, even if the grass is another colour.

Perceptual defence

People tend to perceive what they want to perceive and may fail to perceive what they do not wish to perceive e.g., patients may refuse to perceive the truth concerning their illness or injury.

Memory
A mental reconstruction of past events.
Short-term memory is for immediate use e.g. looking at a phone number, then dialling it. *Long-term memory* is a store of information, and can be improved by associative memories (see associative learning). Time is required for the neurological changes resulting in consolidation of memory. Consolidation may be prevented by concussion, resulting in retrograde amnesia, which is loss of memory backwards in time from the time of injury. Mental deterioration and ageing can also result in retrograde amnesia.

Personality
Made up of a collection of behaviour tendencies (traits) of varying degrees e.g. aggression, generosity, ambition.
Two main dimensions are recognized:
1. Extraversion   –   Introversion
   (likes constant   (likes quiet
   excitement)   life)
   Evidence suggests that introverts have a more active ascending reticular system.
2. Neuroticism – Stability
   May be related to activity of the autonomic nervous system.
   Various traits interact within individuals to give a variety of personality types.
   Innate tendencies interact with the environment and experience to produce the personality.

Motivation or drive
Some motivation is physiological e.g. hunger, thirst and sex drives are essential for survival and perpetuation of the species. Drives also exist to seek comfort, security and freedom from pain. Man is a social animal and when the above drives are satisfied he usually seeks the company and respect of others. Still higher motivations are creative e.g. art, music, drama.
Motivations may change dramatically when a person is ill, in pain, or confined to hospital. Therapists can develop the skill to steer the patient's motivation towards rehabilitation and recovery.

Emotion
A subjective experience (feeling).
Emotions such as fear, rage, pleasure correlate highly with physiological states. Evidence suggests that emotions are largely due to activity in various regions of the brain, especially the mid-brain and limbic system. The therapist should be aware that brain damage can result in behavioural aspects of emotion occurring, while the subjective feelings are absent.
Physiological changes are usually produced as a result of emotional experience, but some evidence suggests that production

of the appropriate physiological changes can likewise cause some elements of the correlated emotion e.g. excitement causes release of adrenaline, and injection of adrenaline makes a person more excitable.

SOCIAL PSYCHOLOGY

Humans tend to congregate in groups.

Each group develops norms of behaviour in the way they respond to each other in matters relating to birth, marriage, death, earning a living, feeding and an almost infinite range of activities. Such groups are known as cultures.

Socialization is the process by which the developing child is persuaded to conform to cultural norms by use of rewards (operant conditioning), punishments (avoidance conditioning) and imitation.

Adults who deviate widely from cultural norms usually find that the group exerts sanctions on them in an attempt to persuade them to return to the norm. Continual refusal to respond to such sanctions frequently results in a group decision to ignore the deviant.

Most people like to belong to, and be accepted and respected by a group. Some members emerge as leaders, and fulfil a leadership role which may be aimed at enabling the group to perform a particular group task (e.g. a department superintendent) or a leader may concentrate more on retaining the cohesion of the group (e.g. personnel officer).

Norms of behaviour vary enormously between cultures, so that an aspect of behaviour which is accepted in one culture may cause extreme offence in another culture.

Communication between adults is largely verbal in most cultures, but eye contact, facial expression and bodily gestures are now recognized as playing an extremely important part in 'body language'. Subtle cues from patients may reveal important information to a keen observer. Such cues existed before the development of language.

Stress, tension and anxiety are usually associated with physiological changes in the activity of the autonomic nervous system, adrenal gland secretion, and other chemical changes, such as the balance of intracellular and extracellular sodium. This affects the excitability of nerve fibres. Ability to respond to stress in this manner is a necessary body defence mechanism, but if such changes are prolonged they can contribute to disorders of the heart, digestive system, and other organic structures. Stress is frequently a contributory factor in rheumatoid arthritis.

A patient's reaction to sickness or injury may take the form of depression, regression of behaviour to a more childish disposition, or, if compensation is involved, a determination to avoid full recovery. It is a mistake to assume that such changes are always intentional. They are better regarded as symptoms which can be corrected by operant conditioning and instilling motivation to improvement.

Psychiatric disorders

Details of psychiatric disorders are outside the scope of this chapter, but the International Classification of mental disorders groups them under 3 headings:
1. Psychoses including
   Schizophrenia
   Manic-depressive reactions
   Involutional melancholia
   Paranoia and paranoid states
   Senile and pre-senile psychoses
   Psychosis with cerebral arteriosclerosis
   Alcoholic psychosis
2. Psychoneurotic disorders including
   Anxiety reaction
   Hysterical reaction
   Phobic reaction
   Neurotic depressive reaction
   Obsessive-compulsive reaction
   Various forms of psychoneuroses with somatic symptoms
3. Disorders of character, behaviour and intelligence, including
   Pathological personality
   Immature personality
   Alcoholism, other drug addictions
   Primary childhood behaviour disorders
   Mental deficiency

As the science of neuropsychology advances more behaviour disorders are recognized as having an organic basis in faulty metabolism or nerve function.

FURTHER READING

Argyle, M. (1967) *The Psychology of Interpersonal Behaviour.*
  Harmondsworth: Penguin.
Beard, R. M. (1969) *An Outline of Piaget's Developmental Psychology.*
  London: Routledge & Kegan Paul.
Eysenck, H. J. (1953) *Uses and Abuses of Psychology.* Harmondsworth:
  Penguin.
Eysenck, H. J. (1964) *Sense and Nonsense in Psychology.* Harmondsworth:
  Penguin.
Eysenck, H. J. (1970) *Fact and Fiction in Psychology.* Harmondsworth:
  Penguin.
Gillis, L. (1972) *Human Behaviour in Illness.* London: Faber & Faber.
Hilgard, E. R., Atkinson, R. C & Atkinson, R. Z. (1975) *Introduction to
  Psychology.* London: Harcourt.

Hill, D. A. (1974) *Psychology Teaching*. **2**, 2. Association for the Teaching of Psychology.

Hill, D. A. (1977) *Neurology for Physiotherapists*. 2nd edition, ed. J. Cash, Ch. 22. London: Faber & Faber.

Holding, D. H. (1965) *Principles of Training*. Oxford: Pergamon.

Shakespeare, R. (1975) *The Psychology of Handicap*. London: Methuen.

Sheridan, M. D. (1975) *Children's Developmental Progress*. London: NFER Publishing Co.

Singh, M. M. (1967) *Mental Disorder*. London: Pan.

Wright, D. S. & Taylor, A. (1972) *Introducing Psychology*. Harmondsworth: Penguin.

4. General pathology

CAUSE OF DISEASE

Congenital
1. Genetic
2. Developmental

Infections
1. Bacteria
2. Virus
3. Fungi
4. Parasites

Infection spread by air, ingestion, direct invasion through skin.

Ischaemia

Trauma
1. Fractures
2. Wounds
3. Contusions

Physical agents
1. Temperature
2. Radiation
3. Electric shock
4. Increased/decreased atmospheric pressure

Chemical
1. Accidental/purposeful ingestion
2. Industrial hazards

Stress
1. Physical
2. Mental

Deficiency
1. Mineral
2. Vitamin

Drugs

DEFENCE MECHANISMS OF THE BODY

1. Skin
2. Mucous membranes
3. Antibodies/immunoglobins
4. Leucocytes

Inflammation
Cause see page 34

CHANGES IN ACUTE INFLAMMATION

Vascular changes
1. Initial vasoconstriction
2. Succeeded by vasodilatation
3. Stasis
4. Axial stream broadens
5. Margination of leucocytes

Formation of inflammatory exudate
1. Loss of plasma and plasma proteins into tissues
2. Diapedesis and amoeboid movement of WBC into tissues
3. Chemotaxis to site of injury

WBC – phagocytose bacteria and debris; produce antitoxins
1. Neutrophils – amitosis, phagocytosis
2. Eosinophils – increase in allergic reactions
3. Basophils – contain heparin cf. mast cells
4. Monocytes/histiocytes: remove tissue debris
5. Lymphocytes – later stage inflammation

ISOLATION OF INFLAMMATORY ACTION

Fibrin formation
1. Limits spread of infection
2. Forms 'scaffolding' for repair
3. Forms adhesions

WBC response to inflammation
Tissue macrophages – first line defence
Neutrophils in circulation and tissues – second line defence
Macrophages and monocytes proliferate – third line defence

Spread of infection
1. Lymphatics
2. Blood circulation

SIGNS AND SYMPTOMS OF ACUTE INFLAMMATION

Classical signs
1. Redness
2. Heat
3. Swelling
4. Pain
5. Loss of function

Pathological process
1. Vasodilatation
2. Vasodilatation
3. Inflammatory exudate
4. Tissue damage
5. Oedema/tissue loss

TERMINATION OF ACUTE INFLAMMATION

Resolution – complete restoration of tissue

Involves removal of
1. Inflammatory exudate
2. Fibrin
3. Tissue debris

Suppuration

Due to presence of pyogenic organisms
Leads to formation of pus

Abscess

Cavity produced by tissue destruction
If filled with pus drains to nearest surface, or tracks on fascial
planes

Chronic inflammation – low grade inflammatory response to minor injury

Divisions
1. Chronic inflammation supervening on acute
2. Chronic inflammation *ab initio*

HEALING AND REPAIR

Occurs after
1. Causative microorganisms controlled
2. Inflammatory exudate removed

Events
1. Granulation tissue
2. Scar tissue replaces specialized tissues
3. Repair of bone, skin and blood vessels

CLASSES OF IMMUNOGLOBULINS

Serum antibodies or immunoglobulins are protein related
molecules. They are synthesized in lymphoid tissue from plasma

cells which in turn are formed from B lymphocytes. The classes are IgG, IgM, IgA, IgD, IgE.

Properties of immunoglobulins

IgG
Most abundant 80% of total
Includes antibodies stimulated by infection or artificial immunization
Found in blood and tissues
Low molecular weight allows passage through placenta when combined with antigen i.e. Ag-Ab complex activates complement, opsonin activity and leucocytic chemotaxis
IgG can neutralize exotoxins or viruses and promote phagocytosis

IgN
6% of total
Largest molecular weight in immunoglobin group so found only in blood
Appear very early in response to infection
Present on B lymphocyte cell membrane
Activates complement system, opsonization, and lysis
Not very specific antibodies

IgA
3% of total
Large molecule
Found in internal and external body fluids
Protects mucous membranes

IgD and IgE
0.002% of total
Both large molecules
IgD function not known, found on B lymphocytes
IgE attaches to mast cells and on contact with antigen releases histamine and serotonin
Produces allergic response and the hypersensitive anaphylactic response

ANTIBODY REACTIONS WITH ANTIGENS

1. Precipitation, a growing lattice of Ag-Ab reactions which may fall out of blood as a precipitate
2. Agglutination, linkage of adjacent antibody cells
3. Neutralization, antibody-toxin neutralizing complex
4. Complement system (see p. 38)

LYMPHOID TISSUE

Lymphocytes, plasma cells, and macrophages constitute lymphoid tissue. Lymphocytes are classified as B lymphocytes (originating from bone marrow processes) and T lymphocytes (thymus originating)

B lymphocytes
1. Have membrane bound IgM and IgM
2. Form plasma cells
3. Produce 'memory' cells for specific antigen immunity
4. Divide into clones of cells
5. Promote humoral antibody formation

T lymphocytes
1. Concerned with cell mediated responses
2. Cell membrane bound IgM
3. Release lymphokines – attract and retain macrophages to the site of infection

Co-operation between T and B cells
1. Antigens attach to surface receptor sites on T cell
2. The Ag-Ab complex is released from T cells
3. Macrophages pick up Ag-Ab complex and present it to B cell to destroy

COMPLEMENT SYSTEM

A complex system involved in the body's primary response to an antigen, producing an amplifying cascade of reactions, leading to cell death of pathogenic micro-organisms.
Activated in two ways – classical and alternative:

Classical mode
Activated by IgG or IgM complexes – recognition unit C2, C3 and C4 form an activation unit.
The activation unit complexes with C5, C6, C7, C8 and C9 to form a membrane attack unit.
Cell membrane lysis then takes place.

Alternative mode
Activated by endotoxins or IgA.
C3 and C5 form the activation unit and complex with C6–C9 to form the cell membrane attack unit.

IMMUNITY

Acquired or innate:

Acquired
'Learned' specific immunity against an individual invading agent, begins shortly after birth
Naturally acquired active immunity – by producing antibodies in response to infection e.g. chicken pox
Naturally acquired passive immunity – by passage of antibodies from an immunized donor to a recipient
Artificially acquired active immunity – vaccines
Artificially acquired passive immunity – immune serum

Innate
Protective mechanisms inherent at birth
Mechanisms involved are – leucocytes, the fixed and wandering cells of the reticulo-endothelial system, enzymes, acids and lysozyme.

HAEMORRHAGE

Causes
1. Tissue injuries
2. Pregnancy
3. Childbirth
4. Ulcers
5. Varicose veins
6. Aneurysms

Effects
1. Loss of blood
2. Rise in heart rate
3. Fall in BP

Haemostasis and clotting
1. Vasoconstriction
2. Thromboplastin formation
3. Conversion of prothrombin to thrombin
4. Conversion of fibrinogen to fibrin

SHOCK

Signs and symptoms
1. Pallor
2. Coldness
3. Sweating
4. Nausea/vomiting
5. Loss of consciousness

Caused by reduced cardiac output due to
1. Acute heart failure
2. Oligaemia
3. Pulmonary embolism
4. Infection
5. Anaphylaxis
6. Vasovagal attack

Principles of treatment
1. Lie flat
2. Maintain airway and cardiac output
3. Nothing by mouth if unconscious
4. Call for medical help

OEDEMA

An accumulation of excess fluid in tissue spaces.

Mechanism of oedema formation
1. Venous congestion
2. Lymphatic obstruction
3. Hypoproteinaemia
4. Increased capillary permeability
5. Sodium retention
6. Trauma
7. Paralysis
8. Muscle disuse

Principles of treatment
1. Remove cause if possible
2. Increase absorption of fluid by lymphatics
3. Mobilize joints
4. Strengthen muscle
5. Regain normal function

COAGULATION OF BLOOD

When a blood vessel is damaged two responses occur:
1. Vasoconstriction of the damaged vessel to stop blood loss
2. Formation of a blood clot to plug the damaged vessel, this occurs in three general stages
   Stage 1: formation or release of thromboplastin
   Stage 2: conversion of prothrombin into thrombin (in the presence of thromboplastin)
   Stage 3: thrombin catalyses the conversion of fibrinogen into fibrin

Fibrin forms the blood clot.
Two pathways exist for the production of a blood clot – the extrinsic and intrinsic pathway:

1. Extrinsic pathway begins when the tissues around a blood vessel or the vessel itself is ruptured and tissue thromboplastin is released.
   Tissue thromboplastin reacts with plasma coagulation factors IV, V, VII and X to form extrinsic thromboplastin (stage I).
   Stage 2: prothrombin and factors IV, V, VII and X to form thrombin
   Stage 3: thrombin, fibrinogen and factors IV, XIII form fibrin
2. Intrinsic pathway begins with the roughened surface of a vessel
   Platelets adhere to the vessel wall
   Clumping of platelets causes disintegration and release of platelet coagulation factors Pf_1, Pf_2, Pf_3, Pf_4
   Pf_1–Pf_4 react with factors IV, V, VIII, IX, X, XI and XII to form intrinsic thromboplastin (stage I)
   Stages 2 and 3 are as above in the Extrinsic pathway

Once syneresis has occurred the vessel's repair starts with fibroblasts forming connective tissue 'scaffolding' and new endothelial cells proliferate and restore the lining of the blood vessel.

THROMBUS FORMATION – SIMILAR TO BLOOD CLOT, GRADUALLY OCCLUDES VESSEL

Common sites
1. Coronary aa
2. Cerebral aa
3. Aorta
4. Iliac aa
5. Leg veins

Cause
1. Atheroma
2. Sepsis

Sequence of thrombus
1. Embolus
2. Resolution and recanalization

EMBOLUS – SOURCE OFTEN OBSCURE

Types
1. Thrombus
2. Fat
3. Air
4. Amniotic fluid

Effect is to block blood vessel(s) causing stasis.

DEGENERATION AND NECROSIS

Type	Cause	Tissues affected
1. Cloudy	Toxins, anoxia Inorganic poisons	Heart, liver, kidney
2. Fatty	Toxins, ischaemia Chlorinated hydrocarbons	Heart, liver, kidney
3. Necrosis	Toxins, infarction	All tissues
4. Gangrene	Toxins, ischaemia	Limbs, Lung, intestines

HYPERTROPHY AND HYPERPLASIA

Hypertrophy
1. Increase in cell size
2. Occurs in tissues which cannot reproduce

Hyperplasia
1. Increase in cell numbers
2. Occurs in cells which reproduce

Cause of both
1. Hormones
2. 'Extra work'

ATROPHY

1. Antithesis of hypertrophy and hyperplasia
2. Caused by starvation, ischaemia and disuse

NEOPLASM

Cancer is disordered cell growth.

Cause
1. Genetic
2. Environmental
3. Hormonal
4. Virus
5. Chemical carcinogens
6. Radiation

Spread by
1. Lymphatics
2. Blood
3. Invasive growth

Microscopic appearance
1. Epidermoid carcinoma (skin tissues)
2. Adenocarcinoma (lymphoid tissue)
3. Anaplastic – without parent tissue likeness
4. Differentiated – some parent tissue likeness

Sites
1. Skin
2. Mouth
3. Lung
4. Stomach
5. Breast
6. Uterus

FURTHER READING

Boyd, W. (1971) *Introduction to the Study of Disease*. Philadelphia: Lea & Febiger.
Cotton, R. E. (1983) *Lecture Notes on Pathology*. London: Blackwell.
Hurley, J. V. (1972) *Acute Inflammation*. Edinburgh: Churchill Livingstone.
Ward, F. A. (1977) *Primer of Pathology*. London: Butterworth.

5. Diseases and injuries of the nervous system

HEAD INJURIES

Severity depends on degree of brain damage sustained, not on the extent of the skull fracture.

Common causes
1. Road traffic accidents
2. Industrial accidents
3. Domestic accidents

Males more commonly involved than females, with the highest incidence in the 15–34 age group.

Brain injury results from
1. Deceleration force e.g. when the head is suddenly stopped by the dashboard in a road traffic accident
2. Acceleration force e.g. knock-out blow
3. Depressed fracture or penetrating wound of skull

Primary brain damage
1. Confusion and laceration at site of blow
2. Brain cell damage and diffuse axonal disruption by rotational and deceleration forces

This results from external forces on the skull which is rigid, but has an irregular internal contour, and on the brain which is not rigid, but lacks compressibility. Confusion is therefore common in frontal and temporal lobes.

   This diffuse structural damage necessarily leads to diverse neurological signs and symptoms. The severity of primary brain damage which may range between minimal and extreme may be classified by:
1. Duration and level of coma
2. Length of post-traumatic amnesia

Brain damage may be measured by:
1. Computer tomography
2. Nuclear magnetic resonance
3. Electrophysiological techniques

Secondary brain damage
The consequence of a complication which is potentially preventable or reversable with treatment.
May arise from:
1. Intracranial factors
    (i) Intracranial haematoma
    (ii) Subdural haematoma
    (iii) Subarachnoid haemorrhage
2. Cerebral oedema or swelling
3. Infection
4. Cerebral hypoxia from
    (i) Damage to respiratory centre
    (ii) Direct trauma to thorax and lungs
    (iii) Hypotension
    (iv) Use of depressant drugs e.g. morphine

Mechanism of brain damage from hypoxia

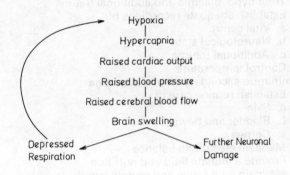

Prognosis
Physical factors influencing prognosis:
1. Extent and site of brain damage
2. Age of patient
3. Presence of thoracic trauma and respiratory complication
   Recovery following severe head injury is a gradual process and no clear division of stages may be made with any accuracy. However, the following categorization may provide a practical outline:
1. Unconscious stage
2. Subconscious stage
3. Conscious stage

General principles of management of head injuries
To save life:
1. Establish clear airway and adequate ventilation
   Depressed respiration and the presence of additional thoracic trauma or other ventilatory complications may necessitate the use of the following:
   (i) Endotracheal tube
       a. To provide a clear airway
       b. To facilitate clearance of secretions
   (ii) Tracheostomy
        a. To avoid endotracheal tissue damage if the need for (i) (a) and (b) extends beyond 6–7 days
        b. To reduce dead air space
   (iii) Intermittent positive pressure ventilation
         a. To increase respiratory function
         b. To maintain normal blood gases
         Any gas administered to the patient must be warmed and humidified
         All precautions against sepsis must be taken
   (iv) Treat hypovolaemia and additional trauma
   (v) Establish adequate recordings of
       a. Vital centres
       b. Neurological state
       c. Additional trauma
   (vi) Control temperature
2. To minimize secondary effects of trauma
   (i) Establish routine care of
       a. Skin
       b. Bladder and bowel
       c. Cornea
   (ii) Maintain electrolyte balance
   (iii) Provide adequate fluid and nutrition
   (iv) Maintain joint range and muscle length

Unconscious stage

Principles of physiotherapy
1. Maintain clear airway and adequate ventilation by
   (i) Postural drainage within any limitations imposed by raised intracranial pressure and additional trauma
   (ii) Vibration and rib springing
   (iii) Mechanical suction
2. Inhibit development of abnormal muscle tone by
   (i) Reflex inhibiting positioning
   (ii) Passive movement
3. Maintain joint length and muscle length by
   (i) Passive movement
4. Initiate programmes of physical, sensory and social rehabilitation

Subconscious stage

Signs and symptoms
Some or all of the following may be seen:
1. Increasing consciousness
2. Return of cough and swallowing reflexes
3. Exaggerated response to stimuli
4. Restlessness, irritation and confusion
5. Some voluntary movement

Principles of physiotherapy
No list may be given since this stage of recovery is characterized by a wide variety of clinical states. Principles of treatment relate to examination findings and are an extension of those of the unconscious state and merge with those of the conscious state.

Conscious state
Signs and symptoms vary with the severity and site of brain damage. Any neurological dysfunction may be seen and physical problems may often be combined with behavioural ones.

Assessment
See page 52

Principles of physiotherapy
1. Maintain clear airway and adequate ventilation by
   (i) Breathing exercises
   (ii) Postural drainage
   (iii) Encouraging active coughing
2. Maintain joint range and muscle length by
   (i) Passive movement
   (ii) Assisted and active movement
3. Inhibit abnormal patterns of reflex activity by
   (i) Reflex inhibiting positioning
   (ii) Reflex inhibiting movement
   (iii) Use of weight bearing techniques
4. Establish communication – both verbally and non-verbally
5. Increase sensory stimulus by
   (i) Encouraging all general sensory stimuli
   (ii) The specific use of afferent cutaneous stimuli
6. Re-educate normal muscle tone ⎫
7. Re-educate righting and equilibrium reactions ⎬ by:
8. Facilitate voluntary movement ⎭
   (i) Use of functional movement related to developmental sequence
   (ii) Use of weight transference techniques
   (iii) Facilitation of isolated joint movement in a proximal–distal sequence
   (iv) Early re-education of movement in a functional setting

9. Re-educate functional activities by
   (i) Choice and adaptation of activities which do not conflict
       with other principles of treatment
   (ii) Choice and use of aids

Common complications of head injury

1. Psychological
   (i) Cognitive e.g. learning and memory defects
   (ii) Attentional e.g. information processing defects
   (iii) Behavioural changes, inappropriate social responses e.g.
         aggressive responses; physically aggressive action;
         attention seeking behaviour
2. Post-traumatic epilepsy i.e. developing more than 1 week post
   injury – affects 5% of all head injuries. Late stage epilepsy may
   also be seen
3. Myositis ossificans – deposits of bone found in muscles and
   joint structure
4. Ectopic calcification – may be associated with
   (i) Presence of long bone fractures
   (ii) Vigorous stretching of hypertonic muscles

MULTIPLE SCLEROSIS

Disease characterized clinically by a wide variety of signs and
symptoms and pathologically by widespread occurrence in the
nervous system of a patchy demyelination which is followed by
gliosis.

Aetiology
Unknown. Generally more common in cold and temperate
climates. Initial attack frequently between 20–45 years. Some
genetic influence may exist.

Clinical picture
Variable, but often characterized by periods of exacerbation and
remission. Mode of onset is generally rapid development of
symptoms from a single focal lesion of white matter. Overall the
picture is of a progressive disorder with an unpredictable time
scale.
   Infection, trauma, surgery or pregnancy may precipitate an
exacerbation.

Pathology
In areas up to 1 cm in diameter of brain and spinal cord:
1. Inflammation
2. Infiltration of leucocytes and plasma cells
3. Degeneration of myelin
4. Reactive gliosis
5. Sclerosis

Signs and symptoms
Relate to the site of the pathology and any combination of signs and symptoms may co-exist.
1. Motor
    (i) Hyper-reflexia
    (ii) Weakness
    (iii) Spasticity – initially extensor, later flexor
2. Visual
    (i) Retro-bulbar neuritis – leading to
        a. Blurring of vision which may progress to uniocular blindness
        b. Pain on eye movements
    (ii) Diplopia
3. Psychological
    (i) Euphoria
    (ii) Depression
4. Cerebellar
    (i) Nystagmus
    (ii) Tremor
    (iii) Ataxia
    (iv) Alteration of postural tone
    (v) Dysarthria
5. Sensory
    (i) Paraesthesia
    (ii) Proprioceptive loss
6. Urinary
    (i) Frequency
    (ii) Hesitancy
    (iii) Incontinence

Medical treatment
Specific medical treatment awaits understanding of the precise nature of the lesion. Acute exacerbations may be treated by steroids, or less commonly, hyperbaric oxygen. When the diagnosis has been established dietary supplements containing linoleic acid may be advocated.
Symptomatic therapy may be indicated for:
1. Bladder symptoms
    (i) Infections – antibiotics
    (ii) Sphincter disturbance – anticholinergic drugs bladder neck surgery
2. Respiratory infection – antibiotics
3. Depression – antidepressive drugs
4. Increased muscle tone
    (i) Antispasmodic drugs
    (ii) Phenol injections
    (iii) Occasionally, orthopaedic surgery

Assessment
See page 52

Principles of physiotherapy
1. Minimize effects of initial attack and subsequent exacerbations by programmes which treat dominant symptoms (see p. 54)
2. Maintain general mobility and promote function by
    (i) Advice on sleeping, sitting, working positions
    (ii) Instruction in gait and other mobility patterns
    (iii) Advice on choice and use of aids
    (iv) Advice on rest/activity patterns
    (v) Provision of specific home exercise programme
Many physical symptoms may co-exist and treatment programmes must relate to assessment of fundamental barriers to normal movement.

HEMIPLEGIA

Disorder of movement, predominantly of one side of the body arising from damage to the brain, or upper segments of the spinal cord.

Common causes
1. Cerebrovascular disease
2. Space occupying lesions

Cerebrovascular disease

1. Infarction
    (i) Thrombosis
    (ii) Embolus
        a. From heart e.g. myocardial infarction, fibrillation
        b. From atheromatous plaques in other vessels
    Infarction accounts for over 60% of all hemiplegia.

Contributing factors
1. Disease of vessels – atheroma, arteritis
2. Disease of blood – anaemia, polycythaemia
3. Disorders of blood flow – reduced cardiac output e.g. syncope, myocardial infarction, arrhythmia

Onset
Develops over minutes or hours; not generally associated with activity and may occur during sleep.
   Infarction – obstructs the blood supply to the area of the brain producing ischaemia and anoxia with consequent neurological damage.

2. *Haemorrhage*
    (i) From normal vessels
       a. Hypertension
    (ii) From abnormal vessels
       a. Aneurysm
       b. Angioma

Space occupying lesions
1. Tumour
2. Abscess
3. Trauma – see page 44

Symptoms of residual hemiplegia may be found in any lesion affecting the motor cortex or internal capsule.
Degree of damage depends on:
1. Severity of lesion
2. Site of lesion
3. State of collateral circulation
4. Age of patient

Signs and symptoms
Any or all of the following may be found:
1. Altered level of consciousness
2. Disturbance in communication
3. Disturbance in postural tone
4. Loss of voluntary movement
5. Sensory dysfunction
6. Visual disturbance
7. Intellectual impairment
8. Perceptual disorder
9. Incontinence

Assessment
See page 52
   The incidence of hemiplegia from cerebrovascular disease increases with age. Assessment of any co-existing age-related pathology may also be necessary.

Principles of physiotherapy
1. Maintain airway and ensure adequate ventilation by
    (i) Breathing exercises
    (ii) Postural drainage
    (iii) Vibration
    (iv) Assisted coughing
2. Inhibit development of abnormal patterns of reflex activity by
    (i) Reflex inhibiting positioning
    (ii) Reflex inhibiting movement patterns
3. Establish communication – verbally and non-verbally

4. Increase sensory stimulus by
    (i) Weight bearing through limbs
    (ii) Afferent cutaneous stimuli
5. Maintain joint range and muscle length by
    (i) Passive movement
    (ii) Assisted active movement
6. Develop normal tone
7. Develop balance reactions
8. Facilitate voluntary movement
    (i) Functional movement in a development sequence
    (ii) Weight transference techniques
    (iii) Development of isolated joint movements in a proximal to distal sequence
    (iv) Development of the ability to place the limb in space
    (v) Use of afferent stimuli (cutaneous and proprioceptive)
9. Re-educate functional activities by the choice and adaptation of activities of daily living in order that they do not conflict with other principles of treatment

ASSESSMENT OF CENTRAL NERVOUS SYSTEM

Higher centres
1. Consciousness
2. Orientation
3. Mood
4. Memory, attention span
5. Attitude to disability

Communication
1. Receptive state
2. Expressive state

Sensory
1. Cutaneous
    (i) Light touch
    (ii) Pressure
    (iii) Temperature
    (iv) Localization
2. Proprioceptive
3. Visual
    (i) Homonymous hemianopia
    (ii) Diplopia
    (iii) Nystagmus
    (iv) Visual neglect
4. Auditory
5. Perceptive
    (i) Apraxia
    (ii) Agnosia

(iii) Disorders of body image
(iv) Stereognosis

Motor
1. Passive
    (i) Resistance to passive movement
    (ii) Response to quick stretch
    (iii) Range of pain-free movement
2. Involuntary
    (i) Tremor
        a. At rest
        b. Intention
    (ii) Associated reactions on attempted movement
    (iii) Athetosis
    (iv) Ataxia
3. Voluntary
    (i) Ability to support limb against gravity
        a. With effect of gravity minimized
        b. In inhibited range of movement
        c. In full range of movement
    (ii) Ability to control isolated joint movement
        a. In inhibited range of movement
        b. In full range of movement
4. Balance
    (i) Static
    (ii) Dynamic
        a. Sitting
        b. Kneeling
        c. Standing
5. Weight transference
    (i) Rolling
    (ii) Sitting
        a. Lateral
        b. Antero-posterior
    (iii) Kneeling
    (iv) High kneeling
    (v) Upper limbs
    (vi) Standing

Functional
1. Swallowing
2. Continence
    (i) Bladder
    (ii) Bowel
3. Self care
    (i) Feeding
    (ii) Washing
    (iii) Dressing

4. Movement
   (i) In bed
   (ii) Bed to chair
   (iii) Sitting to standing
5. Ambulation
   (i) Flat surfaces
   (ii) Rough ground
   (iii) Stairs
   (iv) In complex and crowded environments
6. Social
   (i) Family
   (ii) Housing
   (iii) Occupation
   (iv) Hobbies
   (v) Lifestyle

General physiotherapy principles of central nervous system lesions

The clinical picture resulting from disease or disability of the central nervous system is generally that of functional impairment. This may arise from one dominant symptom or from the effect of a combination of symptoms. Therapeutic programmes must therefore relate to holistic assessment of the patient's motor state. They must not only reflect basic physiotherapy principles and neurophysiology, but also recognize the time scale over which the changes in the CNS may take place.

Application of sensori-motor learning theories and knowledge of motivational factors are necessary for successful implementation (see p. 26).

Immediate carers, relatives and friends of the patient must be actively involved in all stages of the patient's management.

Symptomatic treatment
Two common symptoms are:
1. Spasticity – increased muscle tone characterized physiologically by increased sensitivity to stretch reflex which is released from central inhibitory influences and physically by increased resistance to passive movement
2. Pain, pyrexia, anxiety and joint contracture may induce increased spasticity

Principles of physiotherapy
1. Inhibition of abnormal reflex activity by
   (i) Reflex inhibiting positioning
   (ii) Reflex inhibiting movement patterns
2. Decrease sensitivity of stretch reflex by
   (i) Cold therapy
   (ii) Use of relaxation techniques

3. Facilitation of normal movement patterns by
    (i) Weight transference techniques
    (ii) Re-education of movement within a developmental
         sequence
    (iii) Re-education of movement within a functional approach
    (iv) Use of bio-feedback techniques

Notes
Dysphasia/aphasia – loss or absence of comprehension or of
expression of spoken or written language symbols. May be:
1. Expressive
2. Receptive
Dysarthria/anarthria – partial or complete paresis of muscles of
articulation often associated with swallowing difficulties.
    Apraxia – inability to carry out purposeful movement in the
absence of motor paralysis, ataxia, sensory loss or a difficulty in
understanding. May be:
1. Ideomotor
2. Dressing
3. Constructional
Agnosia – inability to recognize the significance of a familiar
sensory stimulus in the absence of sensory loss. May be:
1. Visual
2. Auditory
3. Tactile or proprioceptive. May include
    (i) Unilateral neglect – failure to use or acknowledge one side
        of the body
    (ii) Anosognosia – lack of awareness of one side of the body
         or denial of disability

ATAXIA

An inco-ordination or clumsiness of movement resulting from an
inability to control accurately range and precision.

Causes
1. Sensory deficit
2. Cerebellar dysfunction
3. Labyrinthine dysfunction (less common)

1. Sensory ataxia is characterized by
    (i) Proprioceptive cutaneous loss
    (ii) Positive Romberg's sign
    (iii) Loss of fine motor control
2. Cerebellar ataxia is characterized by
    (i) Intention tremor
    (ii) Dysmetria
    (iii) Nystagmus

    (iv) Hypotonia
    (v) Loss of co-ordinate movement

Principles of physiotherapy
1. Develop postural tone ⎫
2. Increase balance responses ⎬ by:
3. Develop co-ordinated movement ⎪
4. Re-educate functional activities ⎭
    (i) Proprioceptive facilitation techniques
    (ii) Afferent cutaneous stimuli
    (iii) Functional activities related to developmental sequence
    (iv) Balance activities
    (v) Frenkel's exercises
    (vi) Use of head weights

POLYNEUROPATHY

Disorder of peripheral nerve function resulting in a flaccid paralysis and, commonly, sensory disturbance. Symptoms are too frequently symmetrically distributed.

Common causes
Many classifications exist:
1. Toxic
    (i) Metals e.g. lead, mercury
    (ii) Drugs, chemicals e.g. isoniozid, streptomycin
2. Deficiency – metabolic and haematological e.g. vitamin B_{12}, diabetes mellitus, chronic alcoholism, folic acid deficiency, porphyria
3. Infective e.g. leprosy, tetanus
4. Post-infective e.g. acute poly-infective – polyradiculoneuropathy (the Guillain-Barré syndrome)

Pathology
Axonal degeneration and/or segmental demyelination.

Signs and symptoms
1. Motor – weakness, paresis often initially distally and progressing proximally. Other patterns may exist
2. Sensory – numbness, paraesthesia of glove and stocking distribution and often accompanied by an unpleasant burning sensation and pain

Medical treatment
1. Directed towards alleviation or cure of basic cause
2. Assisted ventilation if required

Guillain-Barré syndrome

Frequently preceded by a 'flu' like illness. Onset is acute, and deterioration may be rapid, progressing to include not only peripheral muscles, but also those of respiration. Sensory involvement tends to be less marked. Steroids may be given to arrest or reverse the course of the disease.

Assessment of all polyneuropathies

1. Respiration
   - (i) Rate of respiration
   - (ii) Chest expansion
   - (iii) Vital capacity
2. Motor power
3. Sensation
   - (i) Cutaneous
   - (ii) Proprioceptive
4. Joint range
5. Function

Principles of physiotherapy

1. Maintain airway and adequate ventilation by
   - (i) Breathing exercises
   - (ii) Postural drainage, vibration, assisted coughing
   - (iii) Assisted ventilation – see page 92
2. Maintain joint range and muscle length by
   - (i) Passive movement
   - (ii) Positioning and splinting
3. Strengthen affected muscles by
   - (i) Neuromuscular facilitation techniques
   - (ii) Progressive resistance exercises
   - (iii) Equilibrium and righting reactions
   - (iv) Free active exercises
   - (v) Springs and pulleys
   - (vi) Suspension therapy
   - (vii) Afferent cutaneous stimuli
   - (viii) Hydrotherapy
4. Increase sensory awareness by
   - (i) Cutaneous stimulation
   - (ii) Use of alternative sensory pathways e.g. vision
5. Re-educate function by
   - (i) Activities of daily living
   - (ii) Choice and use of aids

FACIAL PALSY (Bell's palsy)

Acute unilateral peripheral lesion of the seventh cranial nerve. Frequently it results from pressure caused by inflammation of the nerve within the facial canal.

Common causes
1. Idiopathic
2. Herpes zoster of geniculate ganglion (Ramsay Hunt syndrome)
3. Middle ear conditions
   (i) Infection
   (ii) Complications of surgery

Signs and symptoms
On affected side:
1. Loss of facial expression
2. Loss of eye closure
3. Loss of ability to purse lips or retract angle of mouth
4. Ballooning of cheek on mastication and respiration
5. Loss of taste of anterior two-thirds of tongue if lesion occurs in proximal part of facial canal

Medical treatment
1. Steroids to minimize swelling in facial canal
2. Analgesics for pain relief

Principles of physiotherapy
Re-education of facial muscles by:
1. Active exercise
2. Neuromuscular facilitation techniques
3. Splinting
4. Care of cornea
Note: 80% of all idiopathic facial palsy recovers within 4 weeks.

PERIPHERAL NERVE INJURIES

Types of injury:

Neuropraxia
1. Loss of conduction without degeneration
2. Nerve conduction possible below lesion
3. Sensory modalities frequently less affected than motor, and autonomic least of all

Prognosis
Good – recovery usual within 6 weeks.

Axonotmesis
1. Disruption of axon, but nerve sheath intact
2. Wallerian degeneration is followed by axons regrowing to own end organs

Prognosis
Good – time scale depends on site of lesion.

Neurotmesis
1. Disruption of axon and nerve sheath
2. Surgery required to approximate nerve sheaths and enable growing axon to reach correct end organ

Prognosis
Variable – functional recovery dependent on axons reaching correct end organs.
In axonotmesis and neurotmesis classical signs of nerve degeneration are seen – clinically and electrically.

Wallerian degeneration
1. Nerve degenerates proximally to nearest node of Ranvier and distally throughout whole length
2. Debris cleared by macrophagic activity
Process takes up to 21 days to complete and is a preparation for regeneration

Nerve regeneration
1. Regenerating axons send out many branches, one of which becomes myelinated and continues to grow down the neural tube
2. Growth rate approximately 1 mm per day
   It occurs unevenly throughout the regeneration period, being initially faster
   Factors influencing rate:
   (i) Age of patient – faster in younger age group
   (ii) Site of lesion – faster when lesion is more proximal to spinal cord
   (iii) Nature of lesion – faster following spontaneous regeneration than following nerve suture

Signs and symptoms
Motor:
1. Flaccid paralysis
2. Muscle wasting
3. Loss of tone and deep reflexes
4. Shortening of unopposed muscle groups
Sensory:
1. Cutaneous loss
2. Proprioceptive loss
Autonomic:
1. Temperature change
2. Loss of sweating
3. Trophic disturbances
   (i) Loss of hair
   (ii) Delayed healing of wounds
   (iii) Brittleness of nails

Assessment
Motor:
  1. Manual muscle testing
  2. Electrical testing
       (i) Nerve conduction testing up to 21 days
       (ii) Strength duration curve after 21 days
Sensory:
  1. Localization of touch
  2. Proprioception
  3. Two point discrimination
  4. Temperature
Autonomic:
  Sweat test – may not be routinely used
Joint movement:
  Range

Principles of physiotherapy
  1. Maintain or increase circulation by
       (i) General activity of limb
       (ii) Massage
       (iii) Elevation
  2. Maintain or restore full range of movement by
       (i) Passive movements
       (ii) Neuromuscular facilitation techniques
       (iii) Free active movement
       (iv) Use of splints
            a. Rest splints
            b. Serial splints
  3. Increase strength in unaffected muscles and affected muscles
     by
       (i) Neuromuscular facilitation techniques
       (ii) Balance and equilibrium reactions
       (iii) Free active exercise
       (iv) Progressive resistance exercise
       (v) Springs and pulleys
       (vi) Suspension
       (vii) Hydrotherapy
  4. Re-educate sensation by
       (i) Heightening sensory awareness
       (ii) Retraining stereognosis
  5. Promote function by
       (i) Use of trick movements
       (ii) Use of lively splints
       (iii) Games and activities

Nerve suture

Necessary to approximate nerve ends following neurotmesis may be:

1. *Primary* – sutured up to 6 hours following trauma, if wound clean
2. *Secondary* – sutured around 3 weeks after trauma. The nerve ends are previously secured to prevent retraction

Postoperative regime

Time	Immobilization	Principles of physiotherapy
1–3 weeks	Immobilized in plaster with nerve in shortened position. Limb may be elevated	1. Maintain circulation 2. Encourage activity in unaffected joints
3–8 weeks	Gradual mobilization avoiding stretch on nerve	as above plus: 3. Increase range of movement within prescribed limits 4. Increase strength in unaffected muscles
8 weeks onwards	Full mobilization	See Principles of physiotherapy p. 60

Individual nerve lesions

Axillary nerve – C5 and 6
Motor supply:
1. Deltoid
2. Teres minor

Sensory supply:
  Skin over deltoid muscle

Deformity:
  Flattening of contour of shoulder

Functional disability:
  Loss of ability to abduct and elevate arm

Common causes:
1. Dislocation of shoulder
2. Fracture of upper end of humerus

Radial nerve – C5, 6, 7, 8, T1
Motor supply:
1. Triceps
2. Anconeus
3. Brachioradialis
4. Extensor carpi radialis longus via posterior interosseous nerve
5. Extensor carpi radialis brevis
6. Supinator
7. All long extensors of fingers

8. Extensor carpi ulnaris
9. Abductor pollicis longus
10. Extensors of thumb

Sensory supply via posterior cutaneous nerve of arm:
1. Posterior aspect of upper arm via lower lateral cutaneous nerve of arm
2. Lateral aspect of upper arm via posterior cutaneous nerve of forearm
3. Posterior aspect of forearm via terminal radial nerve
4. Dorsum of radial side of hand including thumb.

Deformity:
1. Wrist drop
2. Wasting of extensor muscles of forearm

Functional disability:
1. Loss of synergic action of wrist extensors leads to weak flexor grip
2. Inability to place objects on flat surface

Common causes:
1. Pressure in axilla
   (i) Crutches
   (ii) Arm hanging over back of chair
2. Fracture shaft of humerus
3. Trauma at elbow joint

Median nerve – C6, 7, 8, T1

Motor supply:
1. Pronator teres
2. Flexor carpi radialis
3. Palmaris longus
4. Flexor digitorum superficialis
5. Flexor digitorum profundus
6. Flexor pollicis longus
7. Pronator quadratus
8. Abductor pollicus brevis
9. Opponens pollicis
10. Flexor pollicis brevis
11. 1st and 2nd lumbricals

Sensory supply:
1. Palmar aspect of thumb, index, middle and half ring fingers and corresponding palm
2. Dorsum of terminal phalanx of index, middle and half ring fingers

Deformity:
1. Monkey hand – thumb lies in same plane as palm
2. Wasting of thenar eminence
3. Indicating gesture – loss of flexion of index finger and partial loss of flexion of middle finger

Functional disability:
1. Loss of precision grip
2. Loss of kinaesthetic sense of radial side of hand

Common causes:
1. Laceration at wrist
2. Compression in carpal tunnel
3. Trauma at elbow

Ulnar nerve – C8, T1

Motor supply:
1. Flexor carpi ulnaris
2. Medial half flexor digitorum profundus
3. Palmaris brevis
4. Hypothenar muscles
5. Medial two lumbricals
6. Palmar and dorsal interossei
7. Adductor pollicis
8. Flexor pollicis brevis

Sensory supply:
1. Palmar aspect of little finger and half ring finger and corresponding palm
2. Dorsal aspect of little finger and half ring finger

Deformity:
1. Claw hand – hyperextension of 4th and 5th metacarpo-phalangeal joints and flexion of interphalangeal joints
2. Drift of little finger into abduction
3. Wasting of hypothenar eminence and interossei

Functional disability:
1. Loss of power grip
2. Loss of precision movements of fingers

Common causes:
1. Laceration at wrist
2. Trauma at medial epicondyle of elbow

Common peroneal nerve – L4, 5, S1, 2

Motor supply:
1. Biceps – short head
2. Tibialis anterior
3. Extensor digitorum longus
4. Extensor hallucis longus
5. Extensor digitorum brevis via musculocutaneous nerve
6. Peroneus brevis
7. Peroneus longus

Sensory supply:
1. Antero-lateral surface of lower leg
2. Web of first and second toes

Deformity:
1. Loss of anterior muscle bulk giving sharply defined tibial edge
2. Foot drop
Functional disability:
1. High stepping gait
2. Equinovarus position of foot
Common causes – pressure at neck of fibula by:
1. Tight plaster of Paris
2. Trauma at time of fracture

FURTHER READING

Ashworth, B. & Saunders. M. (1985) *Management of Neurological Disorders*. London: Butterworth.
Bach-y-Rita, P. ed. (1980) *Recovery of Function – Theoretical Considerations for Brain Injury*. Bern: Hans Huber.
Bobath, B. (1978) *Adult Hemiplegia – Evaluation and Treatment*. London: Heinemann.
Brook, N. ed. (1984) *Closed Head Injury: Psychological, Social and Family Consequences*. Oxford: Oxford University Press.
Capideo, R. & Maxwell, A. E. ed. (1982) *Multiple Sclerosis*. London: Macmillan.
Carr, J. H. & Shepherd, R. B. (1980) *Physiotherapy in Disorders of the Brain*. London: Heinemann.
Carr, J. H. & Shepherd, R. B. (1982) *A Motor Relearning Programme for Stroke*. London: Heinemann.
Chusid, J. G. & McDonald, J. J. (1977) *Correlative Neuro Anatomy and Functional Neurology*. Oxford: Lange Medical.
Cotton, E. & Kinsman, R. (1983) *Conductive Education for Adult Hemiplegia*. Edinburgh: Churchill Livingstone.
Davis, P. M. (1985) *Steps to Follow – A Guide to the Treatment of Adult Hemiplegia*. Berlin: Springer Verlag.
De Souza, L. H. (1983) The effect of sensation and motivation on regaining motor control following stroke. *Physiotherapy*, **69**, 7, 238–240.
De Souza, L. H. (1984) A different approach to physiotherapy for multiple sclerosis. *Physiotherapy*, **70**, 11, 429–432.
Evans, C. D. ed. (1981) *Rehabilitation after Severe Head Injury*. Edinburgh: Churchill Livingstone.
Goff, B. (1972) The application of recent advances in neurophysiology to Miss M. Rood's concept of neuromuscular facilitation. *Physiotherapy*, **58**, 12, 409.
International Journal of Rehabilitation Medicine (1980) *Symposium on Neuromuscular Disease*, **2**, 116, 142.
Jennett, W. B. & Galbraith, S. (1985) *An Introduction to Neurosurgery*. 4th edition. London: Heinemann.
Lance, J. W. & McLeod, J. G. (1981) A *Physiological Approach to Clinical Neurology*. London: Butterworth.
Lane, R. E. J. (1978) Facilitation of weight transference in the stroke patient. *Physiotherapy*, **64**, 206–264.
McLeod, J., French, E. B. & Munro, J. F. (1974) *Introduction to Clinical Examination*. Edinburgh: Churchill Livingstone.

Medical Research Council (1972) *Aids to the Investigation of Peripheral Nerve Injuries.* London: HMSO.

Mulley, G. P. (1985) *Practical Management of Stroke.* London: Croom Helm.

Payton, O. D., Hirst, S. & Newton, R. A. (1977) *Scientific Bases for Neurophysiological Approaches to Therapeutic Exercise.* Philadelphia: Davis.

Seddan, H. (1975) Surgical Disorders of the Peripheral Nerves. Edinburgh: Churchill Livingstone.

Sutherland, J. M. (1981)*Fundamentals of Neurology.* Lancaster: MTP.

Voss, D. E., Ionta M. K. & Myres B. J. (1985) Proprioceptive neuromuscular facilitation. *Patterns and Techniques.* 3rd edition. London: Harper and Row.

Walton, J. (1983) *Introduction to Clinical Neuroscience.* London: Baillière Tindall.

Walton, J. (1985) *Brain Diseases of the Nervous System.* 9th edition. Oxford: Oxford University Press.

Williams, M. (1979) *Brain Damage – Behaviour and the Mind.* Chichester: Wiley.

6. Skin disorders and burns

SKIN DISEASES

Acne vulgaris

Pathology
1. Increased activity of sebaceous glands
2. Raised sebum production leads to blocked gland ducts
3. Infection occurs
4. Pustules form
5. Area round pustules inflamed
6. Common sites, neck, face, upper back
7. Cause, changes in endocrine activity, diet
8. Occurs at puberty

Principles of physiotherapy
1. Obtain desquamation of skin
2. Increase vascularity
3. Reduce number of micro-organisms
4. Improve general health and hygiene

Methods
1. Teach normal skin care and hygiene
2. UVR dosage E^0
3. Scheme exercises to improve posture and movement
4. Cosmetic preparations for greasy skin
5. Advice on diet

Psoriasis

Pathology
1. Dilatation of capillaries in dermis
2. Oedema of epidermis, leading to:
3. Increased activity of stratum germinosum
4. New cells form horny scales
5. Removal scale reveals pin-point bleeding
6. Sexes equally affected
7. Cause, endocrine metabolic, familial
8. Associated with rheumatoid arthritis

Principles of physiotherapy
In subacute/chronic stage:
1. Remove horny scales
2. Improve general health
3. Allay psychological fears

Methods
1. Coal tar bath/paste
2. UVR
   (i) General suberythemal dose
   (ii) Local E_2^o to remove tough scales
3. Soothing ointment if skin sore

BOILS AND CARBUNCLES

Pathology
1. Infection of hair follicle
2. Pus formation under skin and subcutaneous tissues
3. Pus discharges to surface
4. Cause, friction, constitutional disorder

Principles of physiotherapy
Post-drainage:
1. Encourage drainage of pus
2. Improve general health
3. Advice on prevention of recurrence
Methods:
1. SWD
2. UVR – E_4 to pus area
3. Medical – antibiotics, diet

GRAVITATIONAL ULCER

Pathology
1. Venous stasis, due to varicosities, thrombus, gravity
2. Poor tissue circulation
3. Area indurated
4. High protein content in oedema
5. Skin damaged by minor trauma
6. Ulcers form and become infected
7. Oedema may reduce joint movements
8. Site – near tibial malleolus
9. Examine with magnifying glass
10. Trace ulcer for records

Appearance of ulcer
Floor – red, may contain pus/slough
Lips – hard, red, non-healing
Base around ulcer – erythematous/pigmented

Principles of physiotherapy
1. Improve venous and lymphatic drainage
2. Combat infection
3. Mobilize foot and ankle joints
4. Strengthen muscles of lower leg (muscle pump action)
5. Encourage WB activities in patient
6. Encourage weight reducing programme

Methods
1. Elevation
2. Pressure bandaging
3. Bisgaard massage techniques
4. Faradism-under-pressure
5. UVR
6. Ice cube massage
7. US
8. Passive mobilization
9. Active and resisted exercises
10. Increase daily walking/cycling
11. Advice on care of ulcer and life-style

PRESSURE SORES

Pathology
1. Caused by ischaemia of superficial tissues, due to body weight
2. Shearing forces between tissue planes
3. Examine sore using illuminated magnifying glass
4. Tracings of sore initially and at intervals
Types of sore:
1. Infected
    (i) Dry, hard, black slough
    (ii) Thin, stringy, soft pus
2. Indolent: uninfected, clean, non-healing
3. Clean healing

Principles of physiotherapy
Local:
1. Remove slough and pus
2. Reduce infection
3. Increase tissue resistance to mechanical trauma
4. Improve circulation
5. Increase rate of healing
General:
1. Build up general body resistance
2. Prevent further sores
3. Strengthen postural muscles
4. Teach transfers

Methods
Local:
1. UVR
   (i) To remove slough dosage $E_4^o \times 10$
   (ii) To indolent sore dose E_3^o
   (iii) To healing wound E_2^o + abiotic filter
   (iv) To base area E_1^o
2. Ice cube massage to sore, dosage 5 min
3. 2 hourly turning
General:
1. Postural exercises
2. Transfers
3. General UVR E_1^o
4. Diet and antibiotics

BURNS

Classification
1. Superficial partial thickness
2. Deep partial thickness
3. Full thickness

Effects
1. Shock – loss of proteinous tissue fluid
2. Anaemia
3. Infection
4. Kidney damage,
5. Cardiac failure

Principles of physiotherapy
Medical:
1. Prevent circulatory failure
2. Control infection
3. Improve general health
4. Facilitate healing-graft
Physiotherapy:
1. Prevent contractures
2. Remove oedema
3. Maintain joint range
4. Maintain muscle bulk
5. Improve circulation
6. Prevent respiratory infection
7. Reassure patient

Skin grafts
Types:
1. Full thickness
2. Partial thickness

3. Free grafts
   (i) Split skin
   (ii) Full thickness
4. Flap grafts
   (i) Tubular
   (ii) Fixed base

Special points re: skin grafts
1. Avoid stretching and massage techniques
2. Care in exercise not to cause oedema/haemorrhage under graft
3. Do not disturb skin grafts
4. No direct heat
5. Care using splinting
6. Avoid infecting graft

FURTHER READING

Downie, P. A. (1984) *Textbook of General Medical and Surgical Conditions for Physiotherapists*. London: Faber & Faber.
Forester, A. & Palastanga, N. (1986) *Clayton's Electrotherapy and Actinotherapy*. London: Baillière Tindall.

7. Respiratory and cardiac diseases

IMPORTANT FACTORS FOR CONSIDERATION

Cyanosis
1. Peripheral
2. Central

Apex beat – position.

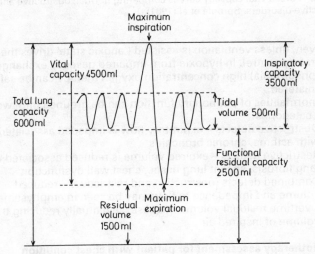

Fig. 7.1 Lung volumes and capacities (numbers for average sized young male adults)

Minute ventilation – tidal volume × respiratory rate per minute.

Diffusion defects – arterial pO_2 and pCO_2 values are relatively normal at rest but decreased with exercise e.g. emphysema.

Blood gas analysis – in the normal resting adult, arterial blood gas values are:

$$pO_2 \ 11.3–14 \text{ kPa}$$
$$pCO_2 \ 4.7–6 \text{ kPa}$$

Oxygen therapy – in chronic hypoxia from hypoventilation (e.g chronic bronchitis) only low concentration oxygen therapy should

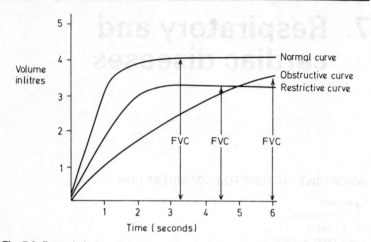

Fig. 7.2 Forced vital capacity curves comparing normal, obstructive and restrictive disorders. Sproule et al (1981).

be given, unless ventilation is assisted ('anoxic state' drives the respiratory centre). In hypoxia from impaired gaseous exchange (e.g. pneumonia) high concentration oxygen therapy can be safely administered.

Abnormalities of pulmonary function can be grouped into two main categories:

1. Obstructive defects – expiratory flow is impeded associated with asthma, chronic bronchitis
2. Restrictive defects – expired volume is reduced associated with lung fibrosis, absent lung tissue, chest wall dysfunction
3. Combined defects (obstructive and restrictive) – reduced volume and impedence to flow may be seen in emphysema. Overtime residual volume increases, eventually reducing the volume of inspired air

Physiotherapy assessment for patient with chest condition
Observation on entry to department/ward.
Patient must then be adequately supported and undressed.

Read notes
Extract relevant information e.g. past medical history, occupation, environment, smoking habits, any heart condition/allergies.

Interrogation
Symptoms – duration
Time/mode of onset of symptoms
General health/activity levels
Progression of condition

Details of:
1. Cough
    (i) When present
    (ii) Unproductive
    (iii) Productive – quality, quantity, odour
    (iv) Any haemoptysis
2. Dyspnoea
    (i) At rest
    (ii) On exertion – note degree/speed of onset
    (iii) Orthopnoea
    (iv) Paroxysmal nocturnal dyspnoea (PND)
3. Presence of pain
    (i) Note details
    (ii) Area, type, intensity
    (iii) Duration, means of relief

Observation
1. General health/appearance
    (i) Weight loss
    (ii) Emaciation
2. Skin colour
    (i) Cyanosis
    (ii) Pallor
3. Shape of thorax
    (i) Barrel
    (ii) Kyphosis/kyphoscoliosis
    (iii) Flattened areas
4. Abnormal respiratory movements
    (i) Unilateral breathing
    (ii) Paradoxical movement
    (iii) Shallow breathing
    (iv) Flail segment
    (v) Accessory muscles
5. Digital clubbing
6. Mediastinal shift denoted by tracheal position

Palpation
1. Tracheal position
2. Chest wall – noting
    (i) Degree/equality of expansion
    (ii) Areas of diminished movement
    (iii) Tenderness
    (iv) Areas of 'blow out'
3. Supraclavicular lymph nodes
    (i) If enlarged infection/malignancy
4. Apex beat position – displacement may indicate
    (i) Enlarged heart
    (ii) Pleural effusion
    (iii) Mediastinal shift

Percussion
1. Dull over collapse/consolidation
2. 'Stoney dull' over pleural effusion
3. Hyper-resonant over pneumothorax, emphysema

Auscultation
1. Audible – wheeze, stridor, bubbling
2. Stethoscopic – vesicular, bronchial, crackles, wheezes, pleural rub

Measurements
1. Vitalograph – FVC; FEV; FE ratio
2. Peak flow
3. Chest expansion – in all areas
4. Range of movement
    (i) Thoracic spine
    (ii) Shoulder joint/girdle
5. Respiratory rate
    (i) At rest
    (ii) On exertion (if practical)
6. Patient's weight
7. Exercise tolerance

Reading X-rays
1. Compare present/past films
2. Observation for abnormalities/worsening
3. Read reports

CHRONIC BRONCHITIS

Definition
A condition with chronic or recurrent increase, above normal, in the volume of mucus secretion, sufficient to cause expectoration, when other localized bronchopulmonary disease is excluded as the source of the increased expectoration.
   When accompanied by widespread bronchospasm, known as chronic obstructive airways disease (COAD).

Aetiology
1. Cold damp climate predisposes
2. Common in cigarette smokers
3. Male incidence higher
4. Manifests in middle age onwards – gradual worsening
5. Greater incidence in dusty occupations, urban habitation
6. Socio-economic factors

Pathological changes
1. Hypertrophy of mucous glands in trachea/bronchi
2. Goblet cells increase, particularly in bronchioles
3. Increased secretions from mucous glands/goblet cells – thick and sticky
4. Mucous membrane thickened
5. Inhaled irritants → bronchospasm
6. Partial obstruction due to (4) and (5)
7. Cilia unable to remove secretions
8. Stagnant secretions → chronic recurrent infection
9. Chronic infection → degeneration – fibrous tissue replaces
   (i) Epithelial lining
   (ii) Some smooth muscle/cartilaginous tissue
10. Fibrous tissue contracts → compensatory emphysema

Clinical features
1. Insidious onset – years
2. Cough
   (i) Initially – lasts several weeks/minimal respite, sputum mucoid, occasionally purulent
   (ii) Later – lasts throughout winter, then all year, sputum quantity increased, periodic acute episodes
   (iii) Advanced – irritating and dry
3. Dyspnoea with or without wheezing
4. Cyanosis (hypoventilation)
5. Exercise tolerance decreases
6. Respiratory movements diminished (apical breathing predominates)
7. Arterial pO_2 falls, pCO_2 rises (often termed as 'blue bloaters' – cyanotic with a barrel chest – poor respiratory drive)

Complications
1. Respiratory failure
2. Cor pulmonale
3. Pneumonia
4. Congestive cardiac failure (CCF)

Principles of physiotherapy
Early stages:
1. Prevent respiratory infection – remove secretions
2. Prevent exacerbations by avoiding predisposing situations
3. Improve breathing control – breathing exercises
4. Chemotherapy where appropriate – bronchodilators, antibiotics, linctus
5. Teach effective coughing
6. Improve thoracic mobility/increase exercise tolerance

Treatment methods
Techniques may include modified postural drainage (PD), vibration/shaking. Later stages – as before but emphasis on:
1. Encouragement of relaxation in all positions
2. Elimination of fear
3. Assisting the patient to understand the condition and his role in the treatment regime
4. Encouraging the maximum use of lung tissue with minimal effort – intermittent positive pressure breathing (IPPB) may be used
5. Mobilizing secretions, vibrations, modified PD
6. Instruction to maintain good postural awareness/control

Acute exacerbation
These patients retain CO_2 and may be drowsy/semi-conscious.
1. Establish adequate ventilation/mobilize secretions
2. IPPB using a face mask – coughing/suction as required
3. Administer low concentration oxygen therapy
4. Bronchodilators may be nebulized
With such patients it is unwise to commence continuous artificial ventilation as 'weaning' is difficult.

EMPHYSEMA

Condition characterized by enlargement of air spaces distal to the terminal bronchioles, accompanied by destructive changes. If generalized, is accompanied by airways obstruction.
Two types:
1. Centrilobular
2. Panlobular
Can occur separately or co-exist.

Causes
1. Localized
    (i) Congenital
    (ii) Compensatory e.g. secondary to resection
    (iii) Partial bronchial occlusion e.g. neoplasm
2. Generalized
    (i) Secondary to chronic lung disease
    (ii) Occupational/excess lung distension e.g. trumpeter
    (iii) Physiological ageing/proteolytic digestion of parenchymal lung tissue

Pathological changes
If from:
1. Partial occlusion/chronic lung disease air flow is obstructed, particularly expiration. Air trapping on expiration, followed by hyper-inflation with inspiration. Walls of terminal airways weaken → breakdown → bullae formation

2. Regular overdistension – atrophy of small airways →
   breakdown → bullae formation
3. Physiological ageing – atrophy of elastic tissue/fibrosis in
   smaller airways. Distension on inspiration, expiration using
   accessory muscles → air trapping → septal breakdown →
   bullae

Signs and symptoms
1. Progressive dyspnoea/orthopnoea
2. Purse-lip breathing common
3. Over use of accessory muscles
4. Barrel chest
5. Diminished respiratory movements
6. Finger clubbing
7. Reduced exercise tolerance
Cough/sputum not particular features.
Often termed 'pink puffers' – breathless but not cyanotic – good
respiratory drive.

Complications
Respiratory failure (slow onset)
Cor pulmonale

Principles of physiotherapy
1. Aid patient in best use of healthy lung tissue
2. Encourage efficient, controlled breathing
3. Encourage relaxation
4. Improve control/co-ordination of respiration during normal
   activity
5. Improve thoracic mobility/general exercise tolerance
6. Prevent respiratory infection – remove secretions
7. Assist patient to understand condition and role in treatment

Treatment methods
1. Local relaxation
2. Basal breathing control
3. Controlled breathing during simple activity
4. Postural control/correction
5. Coughing
6. IPPB (if severe)

BRONCHIAL ASTHMA

Characterized by variable, often paroxsysmal dyspnoea due to
widespread narrowing of peripheral airways – intermittent partial
airways obstruction.
   An attack is caused by increased sensitivity of the smooth muscle
of the airways to a variety of stimuli. Onset may be gradual or
sudden.

Pathological changes
During an attack:
1. Bronchospasm
2. Mucosal oedema
3. Viscid secretion forms plugs in medium/small bronchioles
When a mild attack subsides, chest returns to normal as thick mucus is expectorated.
Following a severe attack → absorption collapse.
Repeated and sustained attacks → hypertrophy of mucous membrane and thickening of all layers of smaller bronchi.

Signs and symptoms of attack
1. May be warning signs e.g. chest tightens
2. Audible wheezing, expiration difficult
3. Dyspnoea
4. Increased respiratory rate
5. Decreased vital capacity
6. Over use of accessory muscles of respiration
7. Distressing unproductive cough
As attack subsides:
1. Bronchospasm ceases
2. Productive cough occurs
3. Patient exhausted
Duration of attack variable (5 min → 24 h).
Over 24 h, status asthmaticus is present.

Principles of physiotherapy
1. Teach patient to understand, control and manage an attack
2. Reassurance – do not show concern over an attack – firm sympathetic handling
3. With a child gain parental co-operation and explain their role to maintain a normal active child
4. Instruction on drug self administration e.g. bronchodilators
5. Prevention of long-term effects from recurrent attacks
6. Instruction on positions of relaxation – to 'ward off an attack'
7. Encourage prolonged relaxed expiration
8. Aid expectoration
9. Control and maintenance of relaxed breathing during everyday activities
10. Maintain thoracic mobility
11. Improve postural defects
12. Encourage normal activities/hobbies

Treatment methods
1. Local/general relaxation – all positions
2. Unilateral/bilateral basal breathing control
3. Relaxed expiration

5. Vibrations/modified PD
5. Expiration/inspiration to counting
6. Strap exercises
7. IPPB – bronchodilators nebulized
8. Assess/progress – vitalograph, peak flow, chest measurements

PNEUMONIA

Acute inflammation of lung parenchyma, commonly bacterial or viral in origin associated with systemic symptoms. Affects chiefly the young child and the elderly.
Two types:
1. Bronchopneumonia – scattered throughout lungs (chiefly basal zones) with local epithelial destruction
2. Lobar pneumonia – localized to airways of one or more lobes (often pleura also)

Predisposing factors
1. Lowered resistance
2. Viral infections
3. Chronic airways obstruction
4. General anaesthesia

Pathological changes
1. Bronchopneumonia
    (i) Inflammatory exudate pus is produced which fills affected alveoli → consolidation or blocks off smaller airways → atelectasis (or both)
    (ii) Resolution follows, but fibrous tissue replaces damaged epithelium
2. Lobar pneumonia
    (i) Vasodilatation → inflammatory exudate/pus which fills alveoli/terminal airways → consolidation
    (ii) Leucocytes/macrophages soften solid exudate, fluid remaining – either re-absorbed or expectorated → resolution if complete, lung → normal

Signs and symptoms
1. Fever, acute onset
2. Dyspnoea worsens with consolidation
3. Reduced respiratory movements
4. Cyanosis if widespread
5. Confused if diffusion defects present
6. Cough – lobar initially dry and painful, with resolution → rusty coloured purulent sputum
    Broncho – purulent from beginning

Principles of physiotherapy
Rest, chemotherapy, oxygen if required
Physiotherapy aims to:
1. Encourage expectoration
2. Regain expansion of area involved
3. Encourage early ambulation to mobilize secretions
4. Maintain full use of healthy lung
5. Increase length of expiration (improve gaseous exchange)
6. Improve general exercise tolerance/thoracic mobility
7. Encourage postural awareness/correction

Treatment methods
1. Coughing, vibrations/shaking
2. Modified PD
3. Humidification
4. Breathing control/relaxed expiration in all areas
5. General mobility exercises
6. IPPB/suction – if severe

Complications
1. Respiratory failure
2. Right heart failure
3. Incomplete resolution

BRONCHIECTASIS

Chronic dilatation of one/several bronchi/bronchioles with
retention of bronchial secretions and persistent infection in affected
lobe/segment. Commonly involves lower lobes.

Causes
Following an infectious disease – thick sputum plugs cause areas of
collapse
Bronchial obstruction
Congenitally weak bronchi
Chronic respiratory infections → fibrosis

Pathological changes
1. Bronchi/bronchioles are totally obstructed
2. Air distal to block gradually absorbed → collapse of distal
   airways
3. Obstructive agent → inflammatory changes in adjacent zone.
   Mucosa loses sensitivity (loss of cilated epithelium) walls
   weaker → fibrosis
   Secretions collect – secondary infection occurs
4. Fibrosis occurs in collapsed areas – contraction follows, which
   produces dilatation of weakened airways immediately proximal
   to blockage

5. Secretions collect in dilatations – 'spill' into adjacent airways → spread infection
6. Inspiratory suction forces, traction, the dilatations – condition worsens

Signs and symptoms
1. Chronic cough, copious purulent sputum
2. Respiratory movements diminished in affected area
3. Reduced vital capacity
4. Haemoptysis
5. Digital clubbing
6. Halitosis
7. Frequently thin/lethargic, postural defects
8. General condition variable e.g.
   (i) 'Ill' – toxic absorption
   (ii) Generally well except for repeated chest infections

Complications
1. From spreading infection/toxic absorption, cerebral/lung abscess, septic emboli
2. Recurrent pneumonia
3. Massive haemoptysis

Management
If condition localized – surgery performed e.g. lobectomy
If generalized – disease controlled by antibiotics/physiotherapy

Medical treatment
Physiotherapy aims to:
1. Remove retained secretions
2. Prevent spread of infection
3. Maintain full function of healthy lung tissue
4. Improve vital capacity, increase respiratory excursion
5. Improve patient's general condition – posture, mobility, vitality
6. Teach self care of chest/respiratory hygiene
7. Encourage patient to lead a normal life, hobbies/sport

Treatment methods
1. Coughing – clapping, vibrations
2. Accurate PD, suitable for home and department
3. Breathing control – all areas
4. Strap exercises
5. General mobility/agility exercises

CARDIAC DISEASE

Ischaemic heart disease
Coronary blood flow is insufficient for the needs of the heart due to narrowing or obstruction of the coronary arteries. Frequently due to atheroma.

Causes of coronary atheroma
Disturbance of lipid transport
Identified 'risk factors' include – high living standards, obesity, smoking, raised blood cholesterol, hypertension, physical inactivity, stress, male > female

Angina pectoris
Clinical syndrome indicating temporary insufficiency of blood flow to myocardium, metabolites accumulate which stimulate nerve endings and cause retrosternal pain with or without radiation.

Generally pain is directly related to physical exertion, eases off in 3–5 min with rest, but it may be precipitated by stress, anger or excitement.

Frequently culminates in myocardial infarction. Coronary artery by-pass graft may be indicated for intractable angina pectoris.

Myocardial infarction
Ischaemia to an area of myocardium → necrosis. Fibrous tissue replaces necrosed area → 'weak spot' (may lead to ventricular aneurysm).

Results in reduced cardiac output/reserve, some degree of heart failure.

Principles of physiotherapy
1. Initially – complete rest/nursing care, relief from pain/shock, oxygen/chemotherapy
   Physiotherapy to prevent complications
2. Later – gradual mobilization within limitations, watch for signs of over-exertion e.g. dyspnoea, tiredness, pallor, chest pain – if present stop treatment – rest
   Check pulse before/after exercise – rate should not rise more than 20 per min and should be normal within 3 min
3. After 6–8 weeks – cardiac class, aimed to
    (i) Strengthen cardiac muscle
   (ii) Increase cardiac output, improve reserve
   (iii) Reassure patient
   (iv) Increase endurance, mobilize/strengthen musculo-skeletal system
4. Give general advice e.g. live within capabilities, take daily exercise, eat regularly but less fats, minimize mental strain

VALVULAR LESIONS

May be acquired due to:
1. Complications of rheumatic fever
2. Degenerative changes superimposed on congenital defects
3. Subacute bacterial endocarditis

Mitral valve most frequently involved.

Valvular defects
1. Stenosis – small orifice, difficulty in opening → back pressure
2. Incompetence – inadequate valve closure, reduced outflow of blood, regurgitation occurs → back pressure
3. Combination of (1) and (2)

Pathological changes
Basically the same whichever valve is affected:
1. Cusps thick/rigid, with calcium deposits on valve margins
2. Chordae tendinae often short, thick and fused together

MITRAL VALVE

Stenosis (more common)

Effects
1. Left ventricle (LV) slightly smaller – less blood enters
2. Raised pressure left atrium (LA) → LA hypertrophy
3. Back pressure in pulmonary circulation
4. Pulmonary congestion/hypertension
5. Back pressure in right ventricle (RV) → RV hypertrophy → heart failure

Signs and symptoms
1. Pulmonary oedema
2. Dyspnoea – graded according to severity
3. Orthopnoea, PND
4. Haemoptysis
5. Malar flush
6. Atrial fibrillation
7. X-ray changes

Incompetence

Effects
1. Ventricular systole → regurgitation LV → LA
2. Reduced cardiac output
3. LA pressure rises → increased LV filling on diastole (Starling's law)
4. → LV hypertrophy → greater incompetence
   Eventually LVF

5. Increased LV filling → greater stroke volume, compensating for reduced cardiac output (BP maintained)
6. Raised LA pressure → pulmonary hypertension (less severe than stenosis)

Signs and symptoms
Early – tiredness, palpitations
Later – enlarged heart, displaced apex beat, exertional dyspnoea, orthopnoea
Much later – pulmonary congestion/oedema, ascites

AORTIC VALVE

Stenosis

Effects
1. Less blood in aorta
2. More blood in LV, pressure rises → LV hypertrophy
3. Reduced cardiac output → reduced coronary circulation
4. Insufficient blood for hypertrophied LV → LVF
5. LVF → raised pulmonary pressure

Signs and symptoms
None until LVF:
1. Angina
2. Dyspnoea

Incompetence (more common)

Effects
Good compensation present, despite large reflux. Cardiac output – normal at rest, slight rise on exercise.
   Compensation for less blood in aorta achieved by:
1. Blood from LA/refluxed blood → raised LV pressure
2. LV stretched → stronger systole → increased stroke volume (cardiac output maintained)
3. Limit of LV hypertrophy reached → atrophy LV → LVF, aortic pressure falls
4. Coronary circulation reduced – insufficient for working muscle → increasing LVF

Signs and symptoms
None until LVF:
1. Exertional dyspnoea, later dyspnoea at rest
2. Angina on effort, later continual pain

TRICUSPID VALVE

Stenosis

Effects
1. Reduced filling RV → small RV
2. More blood right atrium (RA) → RA hypertrophy
3. Back pressure → systemic venous congestion

Signs and symptoms
1. Hepatomegaly, ascites
2. Oedema – sacral, ankles
3. Raised jugular venous pressure

Incompetence

Effects
1. Blood to RA on RV systole, less enters lungs
2. Raised pressure RA, RA stretches → greater diastolic filling RV
3. RV stretches → greater incompetence

Signs and symptoms
As in stenosis but less severe.

PULMONARY VALVE

Disorders almost always congenital.

Stenosis

Effects
1. Resistance to blood flow → RV hypertrophy
2. Pulmonary circulation reduced
3. Less blood passes to LA/systemic circulation

Signs and symptoms
1. Fatigue
2. Exertional dyspnoea → dyspnoea at rest
3. No peripheral cyanosis at rest, may be on exertion

Incompetence
Almost always due to raised pulmonary pressure.
Back pressure to RV makes valve incompetent.
Signs of pulmonary congestion/systemic venous congestion.

CONGENITAL HEART DEFECTS

Possible causes
1. Defective/arrested development in early fetal life
2. Maternal rubella during pregnancy
3. Amniotic adhesions affecting growth symmetry
4. Genetic factors

Disorders may be divided into:
1. *Acyanotic* characterized by
     (i) No peripheral cyanosis
     (ii) No shunting of blood, or left → right shunting
2. *Cyanotic* characterized by
     (i) Peripheral cyanosis
     (ii) Shunting of blood right → left
     (iii) Increased pressure in right heart

Acyanotic conditions
Valvular stenosis
Atrial septal defect (ASD)
Ventricular septal defect (VSD)
Persistent ductus arteriosus (PDA)
Aortic co-arctation

Cyanotic conditions
Tetralogy of Fallot
Transposition of great vessels

Each may occur separately or co-exist.

Common signs and symptoms
1. Acyanotic
     (i) Child thin, small/slow development
     (ii) Exertional dyspnoea
     (iii) Recurrent respiratory infections
     (iv) Excessive fatigue/weakness
     (v) Diarrhoea/vomiting
     (vi) Cyanotic/dyspnoeic attacks
2. Cyanotic
     (i) Central cyanosis
     (ii) Digital clubbing
     (iii) Polycythaemia
     (iv) Squatting position adopted
     (v) RV hypertrophy
     (vi) Fainting, dizziness – cerebral hypoxia
     (vii) Paraesthesia in extremities
In both:
     (i) Heart murmurs
     (ii) Abnormal cardiac shadow

ASD
Foramen ovale remains patent.
Blood passes LA → RA.
Less blood enters aorta → decreased BP.

VSD
Septal maldevelopment → left → right shunting.
More blood passes to lungs/left heart → RV/LV hypertrophy.

PDA
Luctus arteriosus remains patent.
Oxygenated blood diverted from aorta → lungs.
Peripheral blood volume/pressure decreased.

Tetralogy of Fallot
Combination of defects →
  1. RV hypertrophy
  2. Right → left shunt
  3. Less blood in lungs → reduced oxygenation
  4. Mixed blood in aorta
  5. Polycythaemia

FURTHER READING

Amundsen, L. R. (1981) *Cardiac Rehabilitation*. New York: Churchill
    Livingstone.
Brewis, R. A. L. (1985) *Lecture Notes on Respiratory Disease*. Oxford:
    Blackwell Scientific.
Crofton, J. & Douglas, A. (1981) *Respiratory Diseases*. Oxford: Blackwell
    Scientific.
Downie, P. A. (1983) *Cash's Textbook of Chest, Heart and Vascular
    Disorders for Physiotherapists*. London: Faber & Faber.
Flenley, D. C. (1981) *Respiratory Medicine*. London: Baillière Tindall.
Gaskill, D. V. & Webber, B. A. (1980) *The Brompton Hospital Guide to Chest
    Physiotherapy*. London: Blackwell Scientific.
Sproule, B. J., Lynne Davis, P. & Garner, King E. (1981) *Fundamentals of
    Respiratory Disease*. New York: Churchill Livingstone.
Wilkins, R. L., Sheldon, R. L. & Jones, K. S. (1985) *Clinical Assessment in
    Respiratory Care*. St. Louis: Mosby.

8. General surgery, thoracic and cardiac surgery

Common complications
1. Respiratory complications e.g. atelectasis
2. Circulatory complications e.g. phlebothrombosis
3. Haemorrhage
4. Muscle imbalance/atrophy – worse in elderly and debilitated patient
5. Delayed/unhealed wounds
6. Incisional hernia (Fig. 8.1)

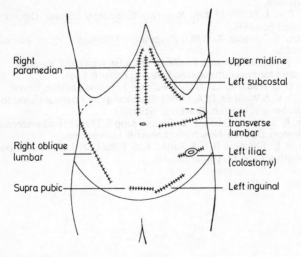

Right paramedian — Upper midline
Left subcostal
Left transverse lumbar
Right oblique lumbar — Left iliac (colostomy)
Supra pubic — Left inguinal

Fig. 8.1 Common abdominal incisions

Physiotherapy

Pre-operative principles
Reassure patient and gain his/her confidence
Brief explanation of what is expected of patient postoperatively

Assess respiratory competence to determine need for:
1. Breathing exercises – stress areas most affected by the surgery
2. Effective coughing
3. Modified postural drainage (PD) – according to patient's condition
4. Foot/leg movements – aimed to aid circulation
5. Postural awareness correction

Postoperative objectives
1. Ensure patient's full co-operation by adequate explanation
2. Remove secretions. Ensure full ventilation of all lung tissue
3. Encourage leg movements. Early ambulation to reduce circulatory complications
4. Ensure correct postural awareness
5. Constant observation for onset of complications

Treatment methods
1. Breathing control – all areas
2. Locate problem areas in chest using
   (i) X-rays
   (ii) Stethoscope
   (iii) Physiotherapist's hands
3. Coughing
   (i) Short sharp blast
   (ii) Prolonged expiration
   (iii) 'Huffing'
4. Aided by – vibrations, humidification or firm pressure over wound
5. Modified PD combined with breathing, coughing, vibrations
6. Active movement of major, lower limb, muscle groups – walk when permitted
7. Posture correction
8. Abdominal muscle contractions – static/active
9. Teach correct lifting of lightweight objects

THORACIC AND CARDIAC SURGERY

Generally surgery is via a thoracotomy or sternotomy incision.

Common operations
Lobectomy
Pneumonectomy
Segmental resection
Pleurectomy/pleuradesis
Valvotomy
Valve replacement
Coronary artery by-pass graft using saphenous vein
Repair of congenital defects

Common complications
1. Lung collapse/consolidation
2. Cardiac arrythmia
3. CO_2 retention
4. Hypoxia
5. Pleural effusion
6. Surgical emphysema
7. Cardiac tamponade
8. Circulatory complications – DVT, emboli
9. Ventilatory/cardiac arrest
10. Restricted arm/trunk movements
11. Haemorrhage

Pre-operative care
Investigations/tests:
1. Chest X-rays
2. Sputum – culture/sensitivity, malignant cell count
3. Blood tests – including gas analysis
4. Dental examination – septic foci treated
5. Respiratory function tests – thoracic excursion, vitalograph, peak flow (vital capacity should be reasonable, if not surgery may create a 'respiratory cripple')
6. Pulse rate, BP

Common prior to thoracic surgery as appropriate:
1. Bronchography, tomography
2. Bronchoscopy to enable observation, biopsy, suction
3. Lung scan – ventilation perfusion scan
4. Mediastinoscopy

Common prior to cardiac surgery as appropriate:
1. Electrocardiography – defects treated when possible, allows for postoperative comparison
2. Apex beat differential count – wide discrepancy indicates left-sided malfunction (commonly left ventricular failure LVF)
3. Cardiac catheterization – results detect degree of damage to each valve
4. May have coronary angiography/Doppler studies determines presence and situation of obstructions

Physiotherapy

Pre-operative assessment
History is taken and examination should include:
1. Shape of thorax
   Acquired/congenital deformity, influence postoperative recovery
   (i) Pectus carinatum/excavatum
   (ii) Barrel chest
   (iii) Kyphosis/scoliosis
   (iv) Asymmetry

2. Respiratory movements
   (i) Amount in each area
   (ii) Symmetry in same area of opposing sides
3. Sputum – note type, quantity, viscosity, colour
4. Indications of cardiopulmonary insufficiency
   (i) Cyanosis
   (ii) Digital clubbing
   (iii) Peripheral oedema
   (iv) Raised jugular venous pressure
   (v) Dyspnoea, orthpnoea, PND
5. Joint movement – note range in
   (i) Thoracic/cervical spine
   (ii) Shoulder girdle/joints
6. Exercise tolerance
   Note speed/distance obtained – on the flat, up slopes/stairs
7. Cerebral function
   Note evidence of CVA cerebral insufficiency and generalized atherosclerosis
   Correlate results of objective tests/special investigations, estimate overall condition
   Inhalation therapy

Pre-operative principles
1. Explain relevance and teach postoperative procedures
   (i) Breathing exercises
   (ii) Coughing
   (iii) Postural awareness
   (iv) Arm, leg, general exercises
2. Encourage breathing awareness/control in all areas of thorax
3. Improve thoracic mobility by
   (i) Trunk/shoulder girdle exercises
   (ii) Bilateral/unilateral rib movements
4. To remove secretions by
   (i) Coughing
   (ii) Modified PD
   (iii) Vibrations/shaking
   (iv) Inhalation therapy
5. Reassurance/basic explanation of patient's role in early and later postoperative period. Explain possibility that patient may return to another ward for 12–24 h – intensive care unit

Postoperative assessment
On returning from theatre prior to treatment the physiotherapist should note:
1. Surgery undertaken – incision used
2. Drainage tubes – number and position, type/quantity of drainage
3. Other tubes present e.g. endotracheal, Ryles, venous/arterial lines

4. BP, temperature, pulse rate
5. Respiration
   (i) Spontaneous – rate/depth
   (ii) Artifical – rate, pressure, volume
6. ECG, blood gases
7. X-ray – compare films
8. Drugs – type, quantity, time of administration
If coincide, analgesics assist treatment.

Postoperative principles
 1. Encourage maximum inspiratory effort – expand all lung tissue
 2. Prevent lung collapse/consolidation by removing secretions
    (i) Coughing
    (ii) Efficient controlled breathing exercises
    (iii) Vibrations/shaking
    (iv) Modified PD
    (v) Suction
    (vi) Alteration in volume/speed of air flow
 3. Prevent circulatory complications by
    (i) General bed mobility
    (ii) Foot/lower limb movements
    (iii) Early ambulation
    (iv) Deep breathing
    A non-extensible webbing bandage tied to foot of bed assists general mobility
 4. To improve maintain thoracic, spinal, shoulder girdle/joint mobility by
    (i) Passive movements (if unconscious)
    (ii) Active assisted/active movement
    (iii) Resisted movement
    (iv) Postural awareness/correction of posture
 5. To increase endurance/exercise tolerance
 6. To enable patient to return to as full and active life as possible

PRINCIPLES OF PHYSIOTHERAPY WHEN PATIENT IS ON A VENTILATOR

1. Chest care
   (i) To prevent infection by removing excess secretions – suction combined with shaking, vibrations, rib springing, manual hyperinflation (bagging)
   (ii) To prevent lung collapse/consolidation by altering rate/depth of respiration – achieved by regular (2 hourly) hyperinflation techniques/forced inflations, regular turning
   (iii) To maintain/reduce viscosity of secretions – if tenacious, saline may be infused into airways

2. Movement and positioning
   Variable according to:
   (i) Reason for artificial ventilation
   (ii) Patient's general condition
   When appropriate the physiotherapist should:
   a. Instruct patient to perform routine maintenance exercises
   b. Perform active assisted/free exercise to maintain joint range, muscle power/length, and aid venous return
   c. Perform passive movements to maintain joint range, muscle length and aid venous return (when patient is paralysed/unconscious)
   d. Position the patient so good posture can be maintained

FURTHER READING

Bain, W. H. & Kennedy W. J. (1975) *The Essentials of Cardiovascular Surgery*. Edinburgh: Churchill Livingstone.

Downie, P. A. (1983) *Cash's Textbook of Chest, Heart and Vascular Disorders for Physiotherapists*. London: Faber & Faber.

Downie, P. A. (1984) *Cash's Textbook of General Medical and Surgical Conditions for Physiotherapists*. London: Faber & Faber.

Ellis, H. & Yorke, C. R. (1982) *Lecture Notes on General Surgery*. Oxford: Blackwell Scientific.

Ellison, N. D. F. (1980) *The Principles and Practice of Surgery for Nurses and Allied Professions*. London: Edward Arnold.

Fleming, J. S. & Braimbridge M. V. (1974) *Lecture Notes on Cardiology*. London: Blackwell Scientific.

Gaskill, D. V. & Webber, B. A. (1980) *The Brompton Hospital Guide to Chest Physiotherapy*. London: Blackwell Scientific.

9. Obstetrics and gynaecology

Complications of pregnancy and their physiotherapy treatment
1. *Breathlessness and/or pulmonary disease*
   Breathing exercises, posture correction and relaxation
2. *Cramp*
   Foot and leg exercises
3. *Oedema of the arms and legs*
   Exercises in elevation
4. *Round ligament pain/sacro-iliac pain*
   Posture correction and relaxation
5. *Costal margin pain*
   Breathing exercises, posture correction and relaxation
6. *Backache*
   Localized, superficial heat, posture correction and relaxation
7. *Varicose veins*
   Foot and leg exercises
8. *Rheumatic, congenital and other heart disease*
   Breathing exercises and relaxation

Other common complications of pregnancy not treated by physiotherapy
1. Abortion – threatened, inevitable, complete, incomplete, missed, recurrent or habitual
2. Ectopic pregnancy
3. Multiple pregnancy
4. Vomiting
5. Heartburn
6. Urgency of micturition and/or stress incontinence
7. Haemorrhoids
8. Cystitis
9. Incompetent cervix
10. Placenta praevia
11. Placental insufficiency
12. Anaemia
13. Pre-eclamptic toxaemia
14. Diabetes
15. Maternal physical abnormalities

ANTENATAL TRAINING

Principles of physiotherapy
To give the pregnant woman the confidence she needs to be in control of her labour by:
1. Giving her a clear understanding of pregnancy and labour
2. Giving advice on posture control and correction
3. Teaching the patient breathing patterns and relaxation techniques which will be of help during pregnancy and labour
4. Giving advice on the role of the husband in labour
5. Preparing her for the postnatal period.

Methods of treatment
1. Classes held in the hospital where the patient is to be delivered
2. Classes held in local health clinics
3. Private tuition

POSTNATAL TRAINING

Principles of physiotherapy
1. To correct posture
2. To restore the correct breathing patterns
3. To restore the tone in the abdominal and pelvic floor muscles
4. To stimulate the circulation
5. To encourage return to normal activities

Methods of treatment
1. A clear verbal explanation is essential as the patients are not ill
2. Posture correction in all positions
3. Diaphragmatic and lateral costal breathing exercises
4. A progressive scheme of abdominal and pelvic floor exercises
5. Advice on lifting, etc.

LABOUR

Signs of labour
1. A 'show' of blood stained mucus
2. Ruptured membranes
3. Regular contractions

Stages of labour
Stage 1: the time taken for the cervix to reach full dilatation. Contractions gradually get stronger and more frequent and some discomfort may be felt in the lumbar region.
Stage 2: passage of the baby through the cervix, along the vaginal canal to outside becoming independent of the mother.
Strong contractions are supplemented by the efforts of the mother.
Stage 3: delivery of the placenta. This usually occurs a short time after the baby is born. Many patients are helped in labour by the administration of various forms of analgesics or anaesthetics.

COMMON GYNAECOLOGICAL CONDITIONS TREATED BY PHYSIOTHERAPY

Prolapse, cystocele, rectocele

Signs and symptoms
1. Discomfort and heaviness in the vulval area
2. Backache
3. Frequency of micturition and/or stress incontinence
4. Occasional pain or burning on micturition

Stress incontinence

Signs and symptoms
1. Loss of urine on exertion
2. Frequency and/or urgency of micturition
3. Backache and/or low abdominal pain
4. Constipation

Causes of prolapse, cystocele, rectocele stress incontinence
Loss of pelvic muscle tone due to:
1. Childbirth
2. Disease
3. Obesity
4. Menopausal changes
5. Senility
6. Failed operations

Principles of physiotherapy
1. To increase pelvic and abdominal muscle tone
2. To restore and increase voluntary pelvic floor control

Treatment
1. Pelvic floor and abdominal exercises, or
2. Pelvic floor faradism and exercises, or
3. Surgery followed by exercises

Pelvic inflammatory disease

Signs and symptoms
1. Diffuse abdominal pain sometimes with swelling
2. Increased vaginal discharge and irritation
3. Backache
4. Increased menstrual flow and dysmenorrhoea
5. Deep dyspareunia
6. Anaemia
7. General lethargy

Causes
1. Pelvic disease
2. Infection following surgery
3. Ruptured ectopic pregnancy or appendix
4. Endometriosis
5. Sexually transmitted diseases
6. Incomplete abortion

Principles of physiotherapy
1. To help reduce infection
2. To relieve pain

Treatment
1. Cross-fire short-wave diathermy
2. Gentle mobilizing exercises
3. Relaxation

Dysmenorrhoea

Signs and symptoms
1. Premenstrual tension
2. Menstrual pain
3. Backache
4. Nausea
5. Vomiting
6. Fainting

Causes
1. Fear and misunderstanding of the menstrual cycle i.e. tension
2. Pelvic inflammatory disease
3. Genital abnormality
4. Pelvic cysts or tumours

Principles of physiotherapy
1. To reduce pain and tension
2. Improve circulation
3. Aid relaxation

Treatment
1. Vigorous exercise to stimulate pelvic circulation
2. Short-wave diathermy if infection is present
3. Relaxation
4. Dilatation and curettage or surgery

COMMON SURGICAL CONDITIONS TREATED BY PHYSIOTHERAPY

Hysterectomy

Sub-total hysterectomy is the removal of the body of the uterus. It is rarely done because of the possibility of cancer of the cervix in later life.

Total hysterectomy is the removal of the uterus and cervix. It may be done in conjunction with a unilateral or bilateral salpingo-oophorectomy when there is disease of the tubes and ovaries.

Wertheim's hysterectomy is performed because of Stage II or III cancer of the cervix and uterus. It is the removal of the ovaries, fallopian tubes, uterus, cervix, upper half of the vagina, parametria and pelvic lymph glands.

Indications for hysterectomy
1. Cancer
2. Dysfunctional bleeding
3. Intermenstrual bleeding
4. Menorrhagia
5. Fibroids

Pelvic floor surgery
1. Pelvic floor repair is performed to correct varying degrees of prolapse.
2. Vaginal hysterectomy is done when there is a procidentia or when uterine disease complicates a lesser form of prolapse.

Indications for pelvic floor surgery
1. Severe stress incontinence
2. Prolapse

Radical vulvectomy

Radical vulvectomy is extensive surgery done for carcinoma of the vulva. It is a block dissection of the vulva, mons veneris, clitoris and perineal tissue. It often involves skin grafting.

Principles of physiotherapy
1. To maintain good respiratory function
2. To maintain circulation
3. To restore abdominal and pelvic floor muscle tone

Treatment
1. Pre-and postoperative localized breathing exercises and coughing
2. Exercises to maintain circulation
3. Exercises to restore abdominal and/or pelvic muscle tone
4. Posture correction
5. Home exercises

FURTHER READING

Bourne, G. (1972) *Pregnancy*. London: Cassell.

Garland, M. D. & Ouixley, J. M. E. (1971) *Obstetrics and Gynaecology for Nurses*. English University Press.

Heardman, H. (1959) *Physiotherapy in Obstetrics and Gynaecology*. Edinburgh: Churchill Livingstone.

Jenkins, D. ed. (1975) *Having a Baby*. Expectant Mothers Service.

Llewellyn Jones, D. (1972) *Fundamentals of Obstetrics and Gynaecology*. London: Faber & Faber.

Mandelstam, D. (1980) *Incontinence and its Management*. London: Croom Helm.

Noble, E. (1982) *Essential Exercises for the Childbearing Year*. London: J. Murray.

Whiteford, B & Polden, M (1984) *Post-natal Exercises*. London: Century.

10. Fractures and orthopaedics

Fractures are discontinuity of bone structure caused by trauma or pathology

CLASSIFICATION

Through normal bone
1. Closed. Skin intact
2. Open (compound). Skin damaged

Fractures may be solitary or multiple.

Through abnormal bone
Pathological

CAUSES

Traumatic
1. Direct force. Soft tissue damage
2. Indirect force
   Rotational – spiral
   Angulatory – transverse
   Compression – often a separate bony fragment
3. Muscular force
   Avulsion of muscle attachment to bone
4. Stress fracture

In cancellous bone, direct force results in a crush fracture.

Pathological
(Force applied insufficient to break normal bone)
1. Congenital
   (i) Osteogenesis imperfecta
   (ii) Osteopetrosis
2. Infective
   (i) Pyogenic osteomyelitis
   (ii) Syphilis

3. Metabolic
   (i) Osteoporosis
   (ii) Osteomalacia
4. Dysplasias
   (i) Paget's disease
   (ii) Simple cyst
   (iii) Fibrous dysplasia
5. Tumours
   (i) Secondary
   (ii) Myeloma
   (iii) Primary

HEALING OF FRACTURES

Tubular bone (compact)
Haematoma
Subperiosteal and endosteal cellular proliferation
Callus formation – soft woven bone
Consolidation of woven bone to compact bone
Remodelling to normal shape

Cancellous bone
Haematoma
Penetration by blood vessels
Proliferation of osteogenic cells from fractured surface
Action of osteoblasts
Formation of intercellular matrix
Calcification

Factors influencing healing of bone
Local
1. Poor vascular supply
2. Inadequate mobilization
3. Infection
4. Interposition of soft tissue
5. Overdistraction

General
1. Osteoporosis
2. Osteomalacia
3. Senility

SYMPTOMS

1. Pain
2. Loss of function

SIGNS

Local
1. Swelling and haemorrhage
2. Deformity
3. Tenderness
4. Abnormal movement
5. Crepitus

General
1. Shock
2. Other injuries
3. Evidence for pathological fracture

RADIOGRAPHS (two views)

Reveal:
1. The exact site
2. Pattern of fracture
3. Degree and direction of displacement

PATTERNS OF FRACTURES

1. Transverse
2. Oblique
3. Spiral
4. Comminuted
5. Compression or crush
6. Greenstick

DISPLACEMENT

1. Tilt or angulation
2. Rotation
3. Overlap
4. Lateral shift
5. Impaction
6. Distraction or avulsion

COMPLICATIONS

1. Local
2. General

Local complications

Bone
1. Delayed union. Union taking longer than expected, but may still occur
2. Non-union. Union will not occur spontaneously
3. Malunion. Bone unites in a deformed position
4. Avascular necrosis. Death of bone following damage to the arterial blood supply
5. Infection

Joints
1. Adhesions
2. Limited joint range
3. Sudeck's atrophy
4. Late traumatic arthritis

Muscle and tendon
1. Tearing of muscle fibres and tendons
2. Avulsion of tendon attachment from bone
3. Post-traumatic tendonitis
4. Muscle wasting
5. Myositis ossificans

Nerve
1. Neuropraxia. Most common
2. Axonotmesis. Where there has been traction
3. Neurotmesis. Rare in closed fractures

Artery
Arterial blood supply may be impaired in both open and closed fractures.
1. Disruption of a major vessel
2. Thrombosis
3. Intimal damage
4. Compression by tissue. Pressure from oedema, bleeding, tight plaster

Features of impaired arterial perfusion
1. Pain
2. Pallor
3. Paraesthesia
4. Pulselessness
5. Paralysis

Complete obstruction of arterial flow for several hours results in gangrene.
If obstruction is incomplete, or transient, severe damage to nerves and muscles may result, e.g. Volkmann's ischaemic contracture.

Skin
1. Primary damage
    (i) Contusion, laceration, crushing and skin loss degloving
2. Secondary damage
    (ii) Fracture blisters, plaster sores, bed sores

Viscera
1. Brain and spinal cord
2. Abdominal organs
3. Thoracic viscera

General complications
1. Venous thrombosis, pulmonary embolism
2. Fat embolism
3. Crush syndrome

TREATMENT OF FRACTURES

Principles of treatment
First aid and reduction
Immobilization
Restoration/perservation of function

Reduction
1. Closed
2. Open. With internal fixation
    (i) Where closed treatment fails
    (ii) When accurate reduction is obligatory
    (iii) In the presence of multiple injury

Immobilization
1. Prevents malunion
2. Limits risk of non-union
3. Relieves pain
Almost without exception, soft tissue injuries take priority over
fractures therefore immoblization should be in a position of
function.

Methods of immobilization
1. Casts or functional bracing
2. Traction (skin or skeletal) can be
    (i) Fixed
    (ii) Balanced or sliding
3. Internal fixation, can include
    (i) Intramedullary nailing
    (ii) Plating
    (iii) Dynamic screw fixation
    (iv) Vertebral rodding

4. External fixation, can include
    (i) Halo-pelvic distraction devices
    (ii) Skeletal pins with an external bar

Physiotherapy in treatment of fractures

Principles of physiotherapy
1. Maintain normal movement and function of non-injured structures
2. Restore normal movement and function as soon as possible of fractured area

Assessment is necessary before and during treatments
1. Record relevant information
2. Read notes and radiographs
3. Discuss with surgeon and ward sister
4. Understand splintage and surgical treatment

Note the following
1. Cause of fracture
2. Other injuries or illnesses
3. Complications
4. Occupation
5. Home situation

Examination
Ask patient about his/her symptoms:
1. Pain
2. Stiffness
3. Function
4. Sensation
Look for:
1. Changes in colour
2. Skin changes
3. Oedema
4. Effusion
5. Muscle wasting
Feel for:
1. Tenderness
2. Local heat
Test:
1. Muscle action
2. Joint range
3. Sensation
4. Respiratory function
5. Functional activities

PRINCIPLES OF PHYSIOTHERAPY

Co-operation with other members of team
1. Surgeon
2. Nurse
3. Occupational therapist
4. Social worker
5. Resettlement officer
6. Family

Explanation and instruction to patient
1. Explain aims of treatment whenever possible
    (i) Joint range to be achieved
    (ii) Muscle power to be regained
    (iii) Function to be restored
2. Teach exercises to be practised
    (i) State frequency
3. Teach functional activities to be practised

Reduce oedema
1. Exercises in elevation
2. Flowtron
3. Ice
4. Deep breathing exercises to assist venous return
5. Support for dependent limb

Maintain respiratory function for patients with
1. History of respiratory disease
2. Injury of thoracic cage
3. Spinal injury
4. Weak or paralysed intercostal and abdominal muscles

Reduce pain of soft tissue by
1. Ice
2. Ultrasound
3. Heat
4. TNS
5. Movement

Period of immobilization
1. Maintain full movement of all joints not splinted
2. Exercise all muscles – isometrically where no movement is allowed
3. Encourage functional activities and independence

Period of mobilization
Re-education of movement:
1. Mobilize still joints
2. Strengthen muscles
3. Restore equilibrium
4. Retrain independence

Suggested techniques – re-education of movement
1. To mobilize joints
    (i) Free exercise
    (ii) Passive mobilization
    (iii) PNF
    (iv) Continuous passive motion
    (v) Suspension therapy
    (vi) Hydrotherapy
2. To strengthen muscle
    (i) PNF straight resistance
    (ii) Repeated contractions
    (iii) Pulleys and weights
    (iv) Spring resistance
    (v) Use of body weight

PHYSIOTHERAPY FOR PATIENTS WITH FRACTURES OF THE UPPER LIMB

Independence activities to be encouraged when in plaster and during period of mobilization
1. Feeding
2. Writing
3. Dressing
4. Toilet
5. Household duties (waterproof covering of plaster for activities involving water)

Exercises for patients to practise when in plaster
Performed in elevation in the presence of oedema.

Hand
1. Flexion and extension of fingers
2. Full flexion of metacarpal phalangeal joints must be maintained
3. Adduction and abduction of fingers
4. Flexion and extension of thumb
5. Opposition of thumb

Shoulder
1. Elevation
2. Adduction in flexion
3. Abduction in flexion
4. Extension
5. Rotation

Elbow
1. Flexion and extension
2. Supination and pronation

Treatment after removal of splintage
Advice to patient:
1. Care of the skin
2. Position of the limb for comfort, especially at night
3. Position of the limb to overcome oedema
4. Activities to be performed
5. Exercises to practise

To overcome pain and discomfort
1. Ice
2. Ultrasound
3. Hydrotherapy
4. Heat

Techniques to re-educate movement
1. Exercises combining movements of all joints and muscles
    (i) PNF patterns
    (ii) Hydrotherapy
2. Movements localized to individual joints
    (i) Free
    (ii) Assisted
    (iii) Passive mobilization where joint stiffness persists
3. Resistance exercises to weak muscle groups using
    (i) Gravity
    (ii) Manually (PNF)
    (iii) Pulleys and weights
    (iv) Springs
    N.B. No resistance should be given distal to fracture until
         fracture is solid
4. Retrain all grips
    (i) Pincer
    (ii) Light
    (iii) Heavy

PHYSIOTHERAPY FOR PATIENTS WITH FRACTURES OF THE LOWER LIMB

Patients immobilized in bed

Maintain extensor tone and prevent flexion contracture of hip and knee
1. Lie flat for definite period each day, prone if possible
2. Isometric exercises for gluteal and quadriceps muscles
3. Active exercises for non-injured and injured leg (if permitted)

Maintain full movement of foot and ankle
1. Adequate foot support for patients on traction, especially for the elderly
2. Active exercises of all movements foot and ankle, particularly for dorsi-flexors of the ankle and flexors of the toe

Maintain good circulation in the leg
1. Vigorous plantar flexion exercises of foot
2. Active exercises of non-injured leg
3. Deep breathing exercises

Check function and positioning of splints and ensure efficiency of movement
1. Thomas splint and Pearson knee piece
2. Fisk splint
3. CPM
4. Split bed

Treatment when splintage removed: patient not ambulant
See techniques for re-education of movement of upper limb.

Exercises for mobilization of lower limb could include
1. Hydrotherapy
2. Free and assisted movement in all planes
   Simple suspension, abduction and adduction of hip (ropes suspended from monkey pole)
   Sliding board, abduction and adduction hip

Knee
   Wedge on pillow under thigh: extension of knee
   Spring resistance, knee extension (spring suspended from monkey chain)
   Prone, flexion and extension of knee

Foot and ankle
   Crook lying, knees to right and left alternately for eversion and inversion of foot
   Spring resistance to plantar flexion (spring suspended from monkey pole)

Treatment when patients are ambulant

Training in independence activities, such as
1. In and out of bed
2. Standing to sitting in chair
3. Dressing
4. Toilet
5. Gait training
6. Steps
7. In and out of car
8. On and off bus

Activities in preparation for return to work e.g.
1. Climbing (bricklayer)
2. Balancing (bricklayer, bus conductor)
3. Lifting (lorry driver)
4. Bending (gardener, housewife)

Gait training
1. Elasticated support in presence of oedema
2. Commence training in pool or parallel bars

Weight bearing depending on union of fracture
1. Non-weight bearing (NWB) on axillary crutches
2. Partial weight bearing (PWB) on axillary/elbow crutches
3. Full weight bearing (WB) gradually discard aid

Progress re-education of movement
1. Exercises to strengthen muscle and mobilize joints (no resistance distal to fracture until solid)
2. Pulleys and weight in PNF patterns
3. Spring resistance
4. PNF straight resistance. Repeated contractions
5. Body weight resistance
6. Passive mobilization techniques where stiffness persists

Balance and equilibrium
1. Various weight bearing exercises
2. Use of wobble board
3. Progress to circuit training

CRUSH INJURIES OF THE HAND

Cause of injury
1. Mostly industrial
2. Heavy machinery
3. Road traffic accidents

Tissues injured can be
1. Skin
2. Blood vessels
3. Nerves
4. Muscles and tendons
5. Bones
6. Joints

Signs and symptoms
1. Swelling
2. Pain
3. Stiffness
4. Motor and sensory loss
5. Loss of function

Intermediate treatment
1. Cleaning and debridement of wound without tourniquet
2. Primary repair of nerve and tendons if wound is clean
3. Reduction and fixation of fractures
4. Repair of skin by suture, graft or flap
5. Application of compression bandage
6. Hand in safe position
7. Arm elevated

Later surgery
1. Reconstruction of finger or thumb
2. Tendon graft
3. Nerve repair
4. Skin graft

Principles of physiotherapy
Preservation of movement is vital
Oedema must be reduced

Intermediate treatment
1. Active movements, all joints in elevation
2. Encourage functional activities

Treatment when bandages are removed
1. Full active movements – with aid of
    (i) Silicone oil
    (ii) Ultrasound
    (iii) Wax
    (iv) Ice
    (v) Contrast bath
    (vi) CPM
2. Grip training

3. Progressive strengthening exercises of all muscles of upper limb
4. Functional activities
5. Pressure garments to reduce oedema
6. Training for home and work

CRUSH INJURIES OF THE CHEST

Frequently associated with other injuries.

Causes of injury
1. Road traffic accidents
2. Industrial injuries

Injuries may include

Bone
1. Ribs
    (i) Usually multiple
    (ii) More than one fracture in each rib
    (iii) Fracture most common at angle of ribs and usually 5th to 9th rib
2. Sternum
3. Spine
4. Clavicle

Soft tissue injuries
1. Lung – puncture wounds or crushing
2. Pleura
3. Trachea or bronchus – rupture
4. Intrathoracic vessels – usually fatal
5. Oesophagus
6. Pericardium
7. Heart – usually fatal

Complications leading to respiratory embarrassment or failure include
1. Flail (stove in) chest which may result in paradoxical breathing
2. Imploding chest (from fractured sternum and clavicle)
3. Airway obstruction
4. Collection of secretions
5. Lung collapse
6. Pneumothorax – often with surgical emphysema
7. Haemothorax
8. Pain

Immediate treatment aims to
1. Maintain clear airway
2. Maintain respiratory efficiency

Clearance of secretions by one of the following
1. Nasotracheal aspiration
2. Endotracheal tube
3. Tracheostomy
4. Physiotherapy. Modified postural drainage, chest shaking, breathing exercises
5. Inhalations (tinc benz)

Maintenance of adequate ventilation by the use of
1. Intermittent positive pressure ventilation
2. Positive and expiratory pressure
3. Physiotherapy – as above

Management of pain
1. Analgesia – avoid respiratory depressants
2. Local anaesthesia
     (i)   Locally into site of rib fracture
     (ii) Regionally by intercostal nerve block
     (iii) Regionally by epidural block
3. TNS
4. Entonox inhalation
5. Intermittent positive pressure ventilation

Rarely are the following operations carried out for fractured ribs
1. Rib traction as an emergency procedure with towel clips
2. Wire suture
3. Intramedullary pin fixation
4. Introduction of Rush nails
5. Pin fixation sometimes to stabilize chest wall

INJURIES OF THE SPINE

Structures which could be injured
1. Spinal column
     (i) Fractures
     (ii) Dislocations
2. Spinal cord/nerve roots
3. Lung, pleura
4. Abdominal viscera
5. Pelvic viscera

Fractured spine

Types of fracture
1. With or without dislocation
2. Compression wedge fracture of vertebral body
3. Burst fracture of vertebral body

Cause of fracture
Trauma – the resultant injury bears a close relationship with the forces sustained:
1. Flexion – force from above
2. Extension – whiplash
3. Rotation – direct blows or falls
4. Vertical compression – falls from a height
5. Muscle avulsion – fractured transverse process due to psoas pull

Pathological:
1. Osteoporosis
2. Tumour

Treatment of stable fractures
1. Rest
2. Early mobilization with or without external splintage

Treatment of unstable fractures
1. Traction (for cervical fractures) – skull tongs
                                      halo vest
2. Bed rest (for lumbar and thoracic fractures)
3. Open reduction and internal fixation)

Physiotherapy for patients on traction or bed rest (where there is no cord involvement)

Cervical spine fractures
1. Movements of legs and lumbar spine
2. Movements of arms but care in elevation to avoid moving cervical spine
3. Isometric contractions of gluteal and quadriceps muscles
4. Deep breathing exercises

Dorsal spine
1. Movements of arms and legs
2. Deep breathing exercises

Lumbar spine
1. Movements of arms
2. Single leg movement
3. Isometric exercises of gluteal and quadriceps muscles

Progression when surgeon permits to
1. Prone, extension exercises
2. Gradually mobilization exercises and ambulation
3. Progressive strengthening exercises of all muscle groups
4. Training in lifting
5. Posture training

Spinal cord lesions
Can be a complete or partial transection.
Resulting in:
1. Paralysis
   (i) Tetraplegia at cervical levels
   (ii) Paraplegia at lower levels
   Can be flaccid or spastic depending on site of lesion
2. Sensory loss (deep and superficial)
3. Incontinence (bowel and bladder)
4. Loss of vaso-motor response, and
5. Sexual function – impotence in the male

Early complications of cord injury
1. General and spinal shock
2. Pain
3. DVT
4. Pulmonary embolism
5. Respiratory failure in high lesions

Complications of paralysis
1. Respiratory impairment (paralysis of intercostals and abdominals)
2. Contractures which are painful
3. Immobility
4. Loss of independence

Other complications
1. Pressure sores
2. Respiratory infection
3. Urinary tract infection
4. Peri-articular ossification – especially of shoulder and hip
5. Depression

Early treatment of spinal cord lesions
1. Introduction of bowel and bladder management
2. Tracheostomy and ventilation for patients with high lesions and respiratory impairment
3. Good bed posture and regular change of position to
   (i) Prevent contractures
   (ii) Minimize spasticity
   (iii) Prevent pressure sores

4. Application of splints to prevent contractures
   Feet supported at 90° with padded foot board
   Metacarpal joints splinted at 90° flexion with interphalangeal
   joints extended and thumb in opposition

Physiotherapy for the acute lesion

Assessment is essential before treatment
Examination of the following:
1. Muscles noting
   - (i) Power
   - (ii) Spasticity
   - (iii) Flaccidity
   - (iv) Muscle imbalance
   - (v) Reflex responses
   - (vi) Muscle shortening
   - (vii) Contractures
2. Joints noting
   - (i) Range
   - (ii) Endfeel
   - (iii) Contractures
3. Skin noting
   - (i) Pressure sites
   - (ii) Trophic changes
4. Respiratory function
   - (i) Test vital capacity
   - (ii) Observe intercostal diaphragmatic and abdominal
     movement and action of accessory breathing muscles
   - (iii) Examine for secretions in the lungs

Treatment
1. Respiratory physiotherapy
2. Passive movements
3. Facilitation of movement as recovery is observed

Physiotherapy for the early ambulant patient
(Adapted to each patient according to level of cord lesion.)

Re-education of movement
1. Inhibitory techniques for muscle spasm
2. Facilitation of muscle action
3. Strengthening muscle

Training in independence
1. Sitting up and lying down
2. Turning over in bed
3. Balance in sitting
4. Dressing

5. Washing
6. Feeding

Training in self care
1. To prevent pressure sores and trauma to skin
2. Methods of relieving pressure

Progression of treatment

Re-education of movement
1. Progressive resistance exercises
2. Mat work
3. Hydrotherapy

Training in independence
1. Transfers to and from wheelchair, car, lavatory, bed, etc.
2. Wheelchair activities
3. Standing from wheelchair
4. Balance in standing
5. Application of caliper
6. Gait training

Training in self care
Bladder and bowel training

Training in preparation for home
1. Involvement of the family in rehabilitation
2. Home visits for short periods initially
3. The occupational therapist will assess and recommend adaptations to home and supply appropriate aids

AMPUTATIONS

Amputation is the ablation of the whole or part of a limb

Amputation may be
1. Traumatic
2. Surgical

Reason for amputation
1. Necrosis following severe peripheral vascular disease
2. To prevent spread of tumours
3. To prevent spread of infection (gas gangrene)
4. Severe multiple compound fractures e.g. crush syndrome
5. Chronic non-union of a fracture
6. Deformity with impaired function
7. Flail limb

Levels of amputation

Lower limb
1. Hind quarter
2. Disarticulation of the hip
3. Mid thigh – most common in elderly with vascular disease
4. Through knee or Gritti Stokes (retaining the patella)
5. Below knee
6. Syme's
7. Toes

Upper limb
1. Forequarter
2. Disarticulation of shoulder
3. Upper arm amputation
4. Mid fore-arm
5. Fingers or thumb

Postoperative management (depending on site of amputation)
1. Wound is drained for 2–3 days
2. Patient is allowed up after 2 or 3 days
3. Application of stump bandage applied
4. Immediate prosthesis applied in few days (lower limb)
5. Permanent prosthesis fitted later

Principles of pre-operative physiotherapy
1. Gain the patient's confidence
2. Assure respiratory function
3. Commence the rehabilitation programme by teaching appropriate exercises

Principles of postoperative physiotherapy

Prevention of contractures
1. Posture and positioning of stump
2. Appropriate exercises

Control oedema
1. Exercises for all muscle groups of stump
2. Stump bandage
3. Regular wearing of prosthesis

Strengthen muscles of
1. Stump
2. Trunk (for double amputees)
3. Arms (for crutch walking)
4. Scapular (for upper limb amputee)

Functional training
Application and care of prosthesis
Lower limb:
1. Mobility
2. Dressing
3. Toilet
Upper limb:
1. Training in use of prosthesis usually undertaken by occupational therapists in special units
2. Preparation for home and work

CORRECTIVE BONE AND JOINT SURGERY

Indications
1. Disabling pain
2. Instability
3. Deformity
4. Loss of function

Types of corrective operations
1. Osteotomy
    (i) Bone divided close to joint
    (ii) Deformity corrected by appropriate technique
    (iii) Internal/external fixation applied
2. Arthroplasty – joint replacement
3. Hemi-arthroplasty – replacement of one articular surface
4. Excision arthroplasty – excision of joint
5. Arthrodesis
    (i) Surgical fusion of joint
    (ii) Internal/external fixation applied

Operation	*Site*	*Postoperative management*
Osteotomy	Femoral Tibial	Early hip and knee movements PWB within few days
Arthroplasty	Hip	Assisted hip movements WB 3–4 days (surgical approach determines position of potential instability)
	Knee	Continuous passive motion 3–4 days then WB
Hemi-arthroplasty	Hip	Assisted hip movements WB 2 days
Excision arthroplasty	Hip	Bed rest with or without traction 3 weeks then mobilize WB with raise
Arthrodesis	Hip Knee	Mobilize adjacent joints PWB gradually progressing to FWB

N.b. These are possible postoperative regimes and are intended only as a guide to management.

Physiotherapy
Important to understand:
1. Nature of operation
2. The available range of prostheses
3. The surgeon's wishes for postoperative management
Treatment includes:
1. Isometric exercises for major muscle groups
2. Movement of all other joints
3. Progression to mobilizing and strengthening exercises
4. Gait training
5. Check leg length
6. Functional training
7. Advice on appropriate care
8. Instilling confidence with activities

SPINAL SURGERY

1. Decompression – through
   (i) Laminectomy
   (ii) Fenestration
2. Fusion

Decompression

Indications
1. Pain
2. Neurological symptoms
   (i) Bladder involvement
   (ii) Muscle weakness or paraesthesia
   (iii) Absent reflexes

Types of operative procedure
1. Partial laminectomy
2. Fenestration (interlaminar approach)
3. Total laminectomy plus fusion

Postoperative treatment
1. Horizontal bed rest for 1 week
2. Gradual mobilization
3. Discharged 2–3 weeks

Physiotherapy
Assess for neurological change throughout postoperative
treatment
First week:
1. Patient horizontal from 3 days to 1 week
2. Breathing exercises
3. Isometric exercise of main muscle groups

4. Leg exercises including straight leg raise
5. Rolling from side to side
6. Prone lying about 5 days, active extension exercises
7. Patient up 5–7 days

Second week onwards
1. Gradual mobilizing exercises including hydrotherapy
2. Progressive exercises for trunk muscles
3. Gradual sitting when stitches removed
4. Instruction in back care

SPINAL FUSION

Surgical fusion of two or more vertebral joints using bone graft or metal plate and screws.

Indications
1. Pain
2. Instability due to
    (i) Fracture
    (ii) Dislocation
    (iii) Structural deformity
    (iv) Spondylolisthesis

Postoperative treatment
Patient horizontal 3–4 weeks
No movements of spine allowed
Up about 4 weeks wearing support

Physiotherapy
Breathing and leg exercises
Gradual ambulation
Function training

DECOMPRESSION

Removal of laminae and any other structures compressing the cord or nerve roots

Indications
Spinal stenosis
Nerve root compression intervertebral foramina
Compression by tumour

Postoperative treatment
As for laminectomy

SOFT TISSUE RELEASE

Indications
1. Contractures
2. Loss of mobility
3. Pain
4. Instability

Types of operation
1. Tendons – tenotomy, repair, elongation, transposition
2. Ligament – reconstruction
3. Capsule – repair, capsulectomy
4. Fascia – fasciotomy

Postoperative management
Passive stretch and active exercises for released structures
Splintage for repaired structures – avoid stretching until instructed

Physiotherapy
Exercises to maintain the increased range
Passive stretching in some instances

TENDON REPAIR

Types of surgery

Transfer
Tendon of a strong muscle released from bone attachment
reinserted on to a bone or into another tendon. Used to
supplement or substitute for the action of a paralysed or weak
muscle.

Graft
A length of tendon (e.g. palmaris longus, plantaris) divided from
donor muscle and sutured to recipient tendon or tendon and bone
to:
1. Make up for loss of tendon substance
2. Lengthen a tendon
3. Replace a damaged tendon which has become scarred or
   adherent

Postoperative treatment
Elevation
Light splintage or compression bandage
Limb in position to avoid overstretch of repaired tendon
Gentle mobilization

Pre-operative physiotherapy
Mobilize the joint(s) over which the tendon will work
Strengthen all muscles of limb

Active exercise of all limb
Explain postoperative treatment

Postoperative physiotherapy
Exercise limb in elevation
Active exercise for all joints not splinted
Splintage removed (always observe carefully activity of repaired tendon):
1. Active exercise all joints
2. DO NOT PUT TENDONS ON FULL STRETCH TILL SURGEON SAYS SO
3. Flex one joint whilst extending the other
For tendon transplant:
1. Train muscle in its new function
2. Encourage normal active movements
3. Functional training
4. Grip training

DEFORMITIES

Classification
1. Congenital or acquired
2. Postural or structural

Congenital deformities
See Table 10.1.

Causes
1. Genetic factor
2. Factors in maternal environment
   (i) Nutrition
   (ii) Infection
   (iii) X-ray irradiation
   (iv) Chemical (drugs, i.e. thalidomide)
   (v) Posture of fetus (i.e. foot deformity)
3. Idiopathic
4. Trauma at birth e.g. fractures, Erb's palsy of arm

Acquired deformities

Postural
No change in tissue
Can be corrected by patient's effort

Causes
1. Weak musculature
2. Debilitating illness
3. Persistent faulty posture
4. Secondary to another deformity, i.e. short leg leading to scoliosis

Table 10.1

Congenital deformity	Description of deformity
Congenital dislocation of hip (CDH)	Dysplasia of acetabulum and femoral head
	Dislocation of femoral head up and backwards
	(8 diagnostic signs)
	Early diagnosis essential
Foot deformities	
1. Talipes equino varus	As name implies
2. Talipes caneovalgus	As name implies
3. Metatarsus varus	As name implies
4. Convex pes valgus (vertical talus)	As name implies
Congenital torticollis	Rotation of head to one side
	Lateral flexion to other side
	Unilateral contraction of sternomastoid
Spina bifida	Three types:
	1. Meningocele
	2. Myelomeningocele
	3. Spina bifida occulta
	Also other associated deformities, i.e. dislocated hip
	hydrocephalus, paraplegia

Treatment	Surgery
Reduction by manipulation Position maintained by splintage	1. After 1 year old Open reduction with removal of inverted lumbus 2. When deformity is established De-rotation osteotomy Salter osteotomy of pelvis Shelf operation Acetabuloplasty 3. In later life Total hip replacement Arthrodesis
Manipulation and splintage to hold over-corrected position	For uncorrected or relapsed feet 1. Soft tissue release 2. Wedge resection of calcaneum and cuboid 3. Calcaneum wedge osteotomy 4. Tendon transplant 5. Arthrodesis
May correct spontaneously	Soft tissue release
Manipulation Splintage	Tendon transfer Osteotomy
Manipulation Stretching of sternomastoid Posture correction	Tenotomy of sternomastoid
Management of paraplegia	Repair of lesion Corrective surgery to hips, knees, feet and spine
Cerebrospinal fluid shunting (Spitz-Holter valve)	

Structural
Structural change in tissue
Cannot be corrected by patient's effort

Causes
1. Muscle imbalance (paralysis)
2. Bony anomalies (hemivertebra)
3. Bone or joint disease i.e. ankylosing spondylitis, Paget's disease
4. Bone growth disorders, Scheuermann's disease
5. Idiopathic

DEFORMITIES OF THE SPINE

Scoliosis
Curvature to one side

Treatment
Splintage:
1. Milwaukee jacket
2. Plaster jacket – Abbott or Risser
3. Halo-pelvic traction
Surgery:
1. Fusion

Kyphosis
Exaggeration of dorsal curve

Treatment
Mainly treatment of underlying cause

Lordosis
Exaggeration of lumbar curve. Nearly always postural or secondary to kyphosis

Treatment
Physiotherapy

DEFORMITIES OF LOWER LIMB

Mostly structural

Table 10.2

Deformity	Treatment
Hip	
Flexion contracture	Soft tissue/splintage/manipulation
Coxa vara	Osteotomy
Knee	
Genu valgus	Osteotomy
Genu varus	Osteotomy
Genu recuvartum	Caliper or possibly osteotomy
Foot	
Pes planus – many causes	Depending on cause
Drop foot	Drop foot splintage
	Physiotherapy
Spasmodic flat foot	Plaster cast up to 3 months
Metatarsalgia	Metatarsal bar or pad
	Physiotherapy
Toes	
Hallux valgus	Kellar's or Mayo's operation
Hallux rigidus	Rockered sole. Kellar's or Mayo's operation or arthrodesis
Hammer toe	Excision and arthrodesis

GROWTH AND EPIPHYSEAL DISORDERS (OSTEOCHONDRITIS)

Cause
Vascular disturbance, ischaemia, trauma

Signs and symptoms
Pain, limitation of movement, muscle wasting, limp (lower limb)

Table 10.3

Lesions	Treatment	Surgery
Perthes' – upper femoral	Splintage to preserve congruity of femoral head in acetabulum	Triplanar osteotomy of femur to replace head in acetabulum
Osgood-Schlatter – tibial tubercle	Rest until symptoms settle. Possible splintage e.g. plaster	
Köhler – tarsal navicular	Rest until symptoms settle Possible splintage e.g. plaster	
Freiberg – 2nd metatarsal	Rest until symptoms settle Possible splintage e.g. plaster	
Sever's – calcaneum	Rest until symptoms settle Possible splintage e.g. plaster	
Scheuermann's – vertebrae bodies	Rest until symptoms settle Possible splintage e.g. plaster	
Kienböck – carpal lunate	Rest until symptoms settle Possible splintage e.g. plaster	
Osteochondritis dissecans knee joint	Rest until symptoms settle Possible splintage e.g. plaster	Fixation or excision of loose body
Slipped upper femoral epiphysis (associated with Frohlick's syndrome)		1. Knowles pins to hold position. Osteotomy of femur when epiphysis fused 2. Denis Dunn operation

Table 10.4 All are common in the elderly. Pathological fractures easily occur

Disorder	Symptoms	Treatment
Osteomalacia Bone atrophy or rickets of elderly. Deficient absorption of calcium	Patient unwell Generalized aching muscles weak and tender May have deformities	Vitamin D (calciferol) Calcium
Osteoporosis Often idiopathic. Can occur after immobilization, steroid treatment, Sudeck's atrophy and other disorders	Symptom free Minimal deformity	Calcium, phosphorus and protein Physical activity
Paget's disease Osteitis deformans slowly progressive Cause unknown	Deformities particularly of upper limb Complications include cardiac failure and sarcoma	Calcitonin

FURTHER READING: FRACTURES

Anderson, M. E. (1972) Physiotherapeutic management of patients on continuous traction. *Physiotherapy*, **18**, 51.

Apley, A. G. (1973) *A System of Orthopaedics and Fractures*. London: Butterworth.

McRae, R. (1984) *Practical Fracture Treatment*. Edinburgh: Churchill Livingstone.

Owen, R. (1972) Indication and contra indication for limb traction. *Physiotherapy*, **18**, 44.

Powell, M. (1972) Application of limb traction and nursing management. *Physiotherapy*, **18**, 46.

Stewart, J. D. M. & Haccett, J. P. (1983) *Traction and Orthopaedic Appliances*. Edinburgh: Churchill Livingstone.

Wilson, J. N. (1982) *Watson-Jones' fractures and joint injuries*. 6th edition. Edinburgh: Churchill Livingstone

FURTHER READING: CRUSH INJURIES OF THE HAND

Boyes, J. H. (1970) *Bunnell's Surgery of the Hand*. 5th edition. Philadelphia: Lippincott.

Gifford, D. (1974) Silicone oil for hand trauma. *Physiotherapy*, **60**, 350.

James, J. I. P. (1970) The assessment and management of the injured hand. *Journal of British Society for Surgery to the Hand*, **1**.

Wynn Parry, C. B. (1976) *Rehabilitation of the Hand*. London: Butterworth.

FURTHER READING: CRUSH INJURIES OF THE CHEST

Gaskell, D. V. & Webb, B. A. (1974) *The Brompton Hospital Guide to Chest Physiotherapy*. London: Blackwell Scientific.
Keen, G. (1975) *Chest injuries*. Bristol: *Wright*.
Seal, P. V. (1974) Analgesia in the treatment of chest injuries. *Physiotherapy*, **60**, 134.
Wilson, J. N. (1982) *Watson-Jones' fractures and joint injuries*. 6th edition. Edinburgh: Churchill Livingstone.

FURTHER READING: INJURIES OF THE SPINE

Bromley, I. (1976) *Tetraplegia and Paraplegia. A guide for Physiotherapists*. Edinburgh: Churchill Livingstone.
Guttman, Sir Ludwig (1973) *Spinal Cord Injuries. Comprehensive Management and Research*. London: Blackwell.
McCay, E., Hollings, E. M. & Nichols, P. J. R. (1969) Problems of living on wheels. A synopsis. *Physiotherapy*, **55**, 447.

FURTHER READING: AMPUTATION

Clarke-Williams, M. J. (1969) The elderly amputee. *Physiotherapy*, **55**, 368.
Crossland, S. A. (1974) Rehabilitation of the below knee amputee using the pre-formed socket. *Physiotherapy*, **60**, 50.
Davies, B. (1973) The lower limb amputee. *Physiotherapy*, **59**, 350.
Lucy, D. (1972) A temporary exercises prosthesis for use following amputation of lower limb. *Physiotherapy*, **58**, 67.
May, D. R. W. & Davis, B. (1974) Gait and the lower limb amputee. *Physiotherapy*, **60**, 166.
Moncur, S. D. (1969) The practical aspect of balance relating to amputees. *Physiotherapy*, **55**, 409.
Murdoch, G. (1969) Balance in the amputee. *Physiotherapy*, **55**, 405.
Verstappen, H. M. Ch., Thursing, C. M. & Mulder, W. J. M. (1972) A new development in powered prosthesis for the upper limb. *Physiotherapy*, **58**, 232.

FURTHER READING: CORRECTIVE BONE AND JOINT SURGERY

Apley, A. G. (1973) *A System of Orthopaedics and Fractures*. London: Butterworth
Benjamin, A. (1969) Double osteotomy for the painful knee in rheumatoid arthritis and osteoarthritis. *Journal of Bone and Joint Surgery*, **513**, 694.
Britain, H. A. & Howard, R. D. C. (1950) Arthrodesis. *Journal of Bone and Joint Surgery*, **32B**, 282.
Downie, P. A. (1984) *Textbook of Orthopaedics & Rheumatology for Physiotherapists*. London: Faber & Faber.
Freeman, M. A. R. F., Swanson, S. A. U. S. & Todd, R. C. (1973) Total replacement of the knee using the Freeman Swanson knee prosthesis. *Clinical Orthopaedics*, **94**, 153.

Jackson, J. B. Waugh, W. G. & Green J. P. (1969) High tibial osteology for osteoarthritis of the knee. *Journal of Bone and Joint Surgery*, **51b** 1, 88.

McIntosh, D. L. (1972) The use of hemiarthroplasty prosthesis for advanced osteoarthritis and rheumatoid arthritis of knee. *Journal of Bone and Joint Surgery*, **54B**, 244.

Newman, P. H. (1973) Surgical treatment for de-rangement of the lumbar spine. *Journal of Bone and Joint Surgery*, **55B**, 7.

Schatzker, J. & Pennel, G. F. (1975) Spinal stenosis. A cause of cauda equina compression. *Journal of Bone and Joint Surgery*, **50B**, 606.

Smillie, I. S. (1975) *Injuries of the Knee Joint*. Edinburgh: Churchill Livingstone.

FURTHER READING: TENDON REPAIR

Boyes, J. H. (1970) *Bunnell's Surgery of the Hand*. Philadelphia: Lippincott.

Wynn Parry, C. B. (1976) *Rehabilitation of the Hand*. London: Butterworth.

FURTHER READING: DEFORMITIES

Cane, F. (1969) Walking training of the young child with myelomeningocele. *Physiotherapy*, **55**, 3.22.

Eckstein, H. B. (1977) Spina bifida. The overall problem. *Physiotherapy*, **63**, 182.

Gaskell, D. V. (1974) Physiotherapy for scoliotic patients in respiratory failure. *Physiotherapy*, **60**, 71.

James, J. I. P. (1967) *Scoliosis*. Edinburgh: Livingstone.

Kapila, J. (1977) Primary treatment of spina bifida. *Physiotherapy*, **63**, 184.

Kennedy, J. M. (1974) *Orthopaedic splints and Appliances*. London: Ballière.

Madden, B. K. (1977) Orthopaedic aspects of spina bifida. *Physiotherapy*, **63**, 186.

Manning, C. W. (1967–68) Surgical background to coliosis. *Journal of the Royal College of Physicians*, **2**, 77.

Manning, C. W. (1974) Scoliosis. *Physiotherapy*, **60**, 9.

Powell, M. (1986) *Orthopaedic Nursing and Rehabilitation*. 9th edition. Edinburgh: Churchill Livingstone.

Sharrad, W. J. W., Zachary, R. B., Lorber, J. & Bruce, A. M. (1963) A controlled trial of immediate and delayed closure of spina bifida cyctica. *Archives of Diseases in Childhood*, **36**, 16.

Sharrad, W. J. W. (1964) Posterior ilio psoas transplantation in the treatment of paralytic dislocation of the hip in children with myelomeningocele. *Journal of Bone and Joint Surgery*, **46B**, 426.

Sharrad, W. J. W. (1971) *Paediatric Orthopaedics and Fractures*. Edinburgh: Blackwell Scientific Publications.

Taylor, J. F., Oyemade, G. A. & Shaw, E. (1976) Primary treatment of rigid congenital T.E.V. *Physiotherapy*, **62**, 89.

Walton, A. (1969) Treatment of the infant and young child with myelomeningocele. *Physiotherapy*, **55**, 315.

FURTHER READING: GROWTH AND EPIPHYSEAL DISORDERS

Adley, A. G. (1976) *A System of Orthopaedics and Fractures*. London: Butterworth.
Barry, H. C. (1969) *Paget's Disease of Bone*. Edinburgh: Livingstone.
Duthie, R. B. & Ferguson, A. B. (1973) *Mercer's Orthopaedic Surgery*. London: Edward Arnold.

11. Soft tissue injuries and sports medicine

The basic aims and means of treatment of recent trauma are the same no matter how the injury is caused. There are, however, certain factors to be considered when dealing with sports injuries.
1. Athletes are not average people
2. Complex psychological effect
3. Specialized rehabilitation
4. Different sports have typical injuries
5. Highly developed muscles waste quickly

Assessment of injury
Based on the same principles as those used by the medical officer, see Adams (1972):
1. To decide aims and methods of treatment
2. To allow accurate recording of progress

Investigation as to occurrence
When? Where? How?
Pain: region, type, time factors

Observation
Soft tissues: contour, swelling
Skin changes: colour, texture, laceration, etc.
Bones and joints: position relative to anatomical normal

Detailed inspection and palpation
Skin: temperature, colour
Pulses
Muscles: wasting, power, range, spasm, laceration
Tendons: attachments, sheath
Bones: changes in position of prominences, depressions, local tenderness
Joints: deformity. True or false movement. Active/passive range comparison
Region of pain in both types of movement
Crepitus
Ligaments: attachments, tests for integrity
Nerves: anaesthesia, paraesthesia

Principles of physiotherapy
A tabulated list prepared at a sports clinic is ideal for reference.
See Steel (1972).
Important points:
1. Regain/maintain joint stability and mobility
2. Regain/maintain muscle function
3. Re-establish co-ordination
4. Maintain general fitness, including cardiorespiratory efficiency
5. Quick return to activity
    (i) Not to the detriment of the patient
    (ii) Not achieved by the use of trick movements

Classification of injury
1. Bone as the primary site of injury (see Fractures p. 100)
2. Joint as the primary site of injury
3. Soft tissue where bone and joint are not the primary site of injury
There may be a combination.

JOINTS AS THE PRIMARY SITE OF INJURY

Structures in and around the joint are concerned with stability and mobility and the balance between the two.

Degrees of displacement
Dislocation: articular surfaces completely displaced
Subluxation: partial separation beyond normal
Sprain: overstretch of a joint with ligamentous damage but the joint returns to normal position

Possible structures affected
Capsule. Capsular ligament. Synovial membrane
Ligaments intra/extracapsular
Tendons and tendon sheaths
Bursae
Non-articular cartilage e.g. menisci
Amount and consistency of synovial fluid in the joint

Dislocation
Most commonly caused by long leverage, occasionally with shallow joints, by approximation of surrounding parts.

Signs and symptoms
1. Tearing sensation
2. Intense pain easing to an ache
3. Abnormality of shape
4. Abnormal movement and/or limitation of movement
5. Muscle spasm
6. Loss of function

Pathological changes
Acute inflammation, subacute, chronic
Inflammatory exudate leading to possibility of fibrous adhesions
Muscle wasting may occur

Assessment
See page 2 and 147

Principles of physiotherapy
1. Reduction
2. Immobilization
3. Maintenance, where movement is permitted
4. Prevent adhesions
5. Early mobilization with weight or stress relieved and within
   limit of pain, but opinions differ
   Progress is made bearing in mind:
   (i) Direction of dislocation
   (ii) Particular precautions necessary for each joint
6. Re-education of functional movement

Possible techniques
1. Cold therapy
2. Immobilization:
   Sling for upper limb. Additional splintage if necessary
   Traction, splintage or bed rest for lower limb
3. Isometric exercises
4. Passive and/or assisted movement within pain free range
5. Accessory movement: must be well taught and supervised
6. Neuromuscular facilitation
7. Active movement with gradual progression
8. Resistance: springs and weights
9. Ultrasound. Short wave diathermy. Infra-red
10. Group therapy for functional activity once full range is obtained

Complications
1. Fractures
2. Periosteal involvement
3. Capsulitis
4. Synovitis
5. Injury to nerves. Stretch or compression
6. Injury to blood vessels
7. Ischaemia
8. Skin or subcutaneous tissue involvement
9. Limitation of range
10. Abnormal movement patterns
    Gravitational swelling may occur in the limb involved if
    preventative measures are not explained and implemented

Subluxation
The principles of treatment are the same but with immediate treatment and quicker progression.

Sprain
Similar but less severe signs and symptoms with occasionally a more localized pain. Ligament and capsular involvement are common.

Principles of physiotherapy
1. Immobilization
2. Reduce inflammation
3. Prevent/control swelling
4. Avoid muscle wasting
5. Avoid formation of fibrous adhesions
6. Maintain full range of movement in joint and in surrounding areas
7. Obtain full functional activity

Frequently affected joints, knee, ankle, wrist.

Knee
Philip Wiles suggests that with a minor sprain there should be only minimal modification of normal activity with avoidance of extra stress positions. Twisting, turning, quick starting and stopping, etc. See Wiles & Sweetman (1965).
Activity should be maintained where possible to avoid atrophy of the quadriceps.

Important to examination
With a complete rupture of the medical ligament, the knee may appear stable in extension, therefore test in varying degrees of flexion.

Signs and symptoms
1. Pain – acute tenderness over injury site
2. Effusion depending on severity and position
3. Joint instability in severe cases. Tested according to function of ligaments involved
4. Local oedema
5. Inflammatory reaction
6. Difficulty with efficiency of extensor mechanism

Signs and symptoms for sprains in other regions, similar except 6.

Possible techniques
1. Cold therapy
2. Compression
3. Elevation
4. Circulatory exercises in elevation as allowed by splintage

5. Immobilization.
   Compression bandage is often sufficient
   Splint or plaster of Paris in severe cases
6. Isometric exercises for quadriceps
7. Flexion as soon as pain permits. Never forced
8. Ultrasound
9. Frictions. Although frictions produce good results in many
   cases, the upper attachment of medial ligament is an example
   of a situation where they may be contraindicated, the danger
   being Pellegrini-Stieda's disease

The close proximity of structures in and around the knee
determines that if trauma occurs the injury sustained may be
collective e.g O'Donaghue triad. See O'Donaghue (1950).

Meniscus injuries
The medial meniscus is most commonly affected. In function of the
knee an increase in pressure between femur and tibia and including
the menisci occurs during extension. Increase beyond a functional
degree produces a common sign of this injury, namely, 'locking'.
Overlapping of fragments is usually responsible.

Signs and symptoms
1. Difficulty with full extension of knee
2. Joint occasionally 'locks' on slight flexion
3. Rotation is absent in last few degrees of extension
4. Pain at joint level
5. Traumatic synovitis
6. Clicking noise on movement

Complications
1. Limitation of range
2. Instability of joint
3. Muscle wasting or imbalance
4. Osteoarthrosis

Treatment
Surgical: meniscectomy
Follow-up physiotherapy according to the wishes of the surgeon
Time factor is variable

Comment
Personal preference is for early treatment, particularly when
dealing with athletes.
Isometric exercises and some straight leg raising from first
postoperative day. Flexion only commenced after removal of
sutures. Straight leg raising only works the quadriceps statically
with the exception of rectus femoris, and should occupy only a
small part of the exercise time.

A guide for quick assessment with a view to progress to group therapy in the gymnasium
1. No effusion
2. 90° flexion
3. No extensor lag
4. Fairly strong quadriceps. Able to lift a small weight through full range extension
5. Hospital transport not required

Only in extremely rare cases is electrotherapy required.
In combined injuries the treatment of the ligament takes precedence.

Ankle

Treatment
Early use of cold and compression
Severe cases – plaster of Paris
Intermediate stage – contrast bathing
Maurice Ellis sets out a progressed treatment of adequate immobilization associated with contrast bathing and progressive exercises. See Ellis (1972).
The damaged ligament should be in a shortened position when supported.
Grade 1:
Compression. Non-stretch adhesive strapping applied over gamgee tissue
Contrast bathing
Non-weight bearing
Grade 2:
Adhesive stretch strapping and felt pads over local sites
Commence weight bearing
Grade 3:
Adhesive stretch strapping

Exercises
Early stage – do not stretch affected ligaments
Progression – range, strength
A 'wobble board' is ideal for function

Wrist
Immediate use of cold therapy
Support by a metal, plastic or plaster of Paris splint

Principles of treatment
As with other sprains. The tendons and sheaths require additional consideration.

Complications of sprains
1. Oedema
2. Synovitis
3. Periostitis
4. Chronic sprain
5. Osteoarthrosis

Synovitis

The synovial membrane is frequently involved in joint trauma. Continual overstretching, even slight, may result in an inflammatory reaction.

Signs and symptoms
In acute cases the changes are typical of any inflammatory reaction and can be seen after only a short time.
1. Effusion
2. Fluctuating swelling
3. Joint sometimes red
4. Aching-type pain is predominant

Possible techniques
1. Cold therapy
2. Compression
3. Elevation
4. Isometric exercises
5. Circulatory exercises to other joints where possible
6. Progressive active exercise
7. Short wave diathermy is beneficial if a wider circulatory effect is required
8. Ultrasound given marginally

Tenosynovitis

Caused by an irritant which is either internal or external to the membrane.
1. Tearing of fibres of tendon or sheath
2. Repeated stress, even slight
3. Direct blow
4. Repeated pressure
The inflammation may lead to fibrous adhesions.

Signs and symptoms
Variable with cause and structures affected but may include:
1. Pain particularly on movement, acute along the tendon involved
2. Swelling – more often localized
3. Aching in surrounding area
4. 'Grating' feeling on movement

Possible techniques
1. Cold therapy
2. Splintage
   Compression with orthopaedic felt pads and adhesive strapping may be sufficient
3. Ultrasound
4. Short wave diathermy for late developing pain/swelling
5. Frictions after the acute stage
6. Passive stretching
7. Heat treatment for relaxation and circulatory effect
   Some people suggest faradism at the later stage if re-education of individual muscles is required. This is not often necessary but has proved valuable in some cases.

Tennis elbow
Opinions vary as to exact definition. See Adams (1971) and Wiles & Sweetman (1965).

Examples of lesions
Lateral ligament strain
Capsular involvement
Bursitis in the common extensor tendon
Overstretch of fibres of extensor carpi radialis longus or brevis, usually at the musculotendinous junction

Cause
Strong forearm movement, particularly involving pronation and supination associated with strong gripping, is commonly responsible.
Rugby players, golfers, engineers are common sufferers, possibly more so than tennis players.

Signs and symptoms
1. Pain emphasized on forearm movement or pressure
2. Local tenderness
3. Muscle spasm
4. Localized pain but one complication in severe cases is aching and tension of arm and shoulder region

Principles of physiotherapy
Obtain and maintain full range of movement. Pain on movement is likely to persist until range is full.

Possible techniques
Listed by Joan E. Cash (1966) according to actual structure involved:
1. Early stage – cold therapy
2. Supportive sling
3. Ultrasound

4. Short wave diathermy
5. Repeated stretching or manipulation, often in conjunction with an injection of local anaesthetic and hydrocortisone
6. Frictions
7. Heat for more extensive muscle spasm or widespread aching
8. Relaxation
9. Movement – full range must be obtained quickly and then maintained because the tendency to heal in a shortened position may lead to a chronic condition

SOFT TISSUE LESIONS WHERE THE BONE AND JOINT ARE NOT THE PRIMARY SITE OF INJURY

Tearing of muscle tissue
Contusion
Bursitis
Tendon problems (see p. 122)

Tearing of muscle tissue
Common injury in sport.
May be situated:
1. In muscle belly
2. At musculotendinous junction
3. There may be periosteal involvement

Cases of spontaneous trauma frequently occur. Continuous overstrain may be the cause in athletes involved in heavy training programmes. Muscles passing over two joints are frequently affected.

Signs and symptoms
1. Pain, particularly on movement
2. Loss of power
3. Loss of stretch. In conditions where the facial planes between muscles are affected rather than the fibres, stretch may still show a good range
4. Muscle spasm
5. Aching
6. Swelling
7. Haematoma formation may be obvious

Principles of physiotherapy
1. Prevention or reduction of scar tissue
2. Maintenance of muscle length, flexibility and strength. In severe cases of muscle rupture, surgery may be indicated.

Possible techniques
During first 24 h:
1. Cold therapy
2. Compression. More rigid splinting is sometimes required

3. Elevation
   Athletes sometimes feel, particularly with intermuscular
   lesions, that they can 'run it off'. This is not true and will only
   aggravate the situation
   Massage is *contraindicated* and is a common mistake at
   sporting events
4. After the initial 48 h, depending on severity, gentle stretching
   of the muscle is essential. See Gordon (1975)
5. Ultrasound
6. Short wave diathermy

Complications
1. Scar tissue/fibrous formation which limit muscle function
2. Myositis ossificans. Common site, quadriceps
3. Further tearing of surrounding tissue
4. Atrophy of damaged or sometimes adjacent muscles
5. Periostitis where damage occurs close to bony attachments

Contusion
A heavy blow is the cause and muscle tissue is crushed
Bleeding may be quite extensive
Common sites: thigh, gluteal region

Signs and symptoms
1. Affected part hard and swollen
2. Haematoma may be obvious after only a short time depending
   on the severity of the force involved
3. Restricted movement
4. Painful movement
5. Inflammation
6. Spasm in surrounding muscles

Principles of physiotherapy
1. Dispersion of haematoma with minimal scar formation
2. To maintain flexibility, elasticity and strength of the muscle

Possible techniques
1. Cold therapy
2. Compression. In lower thigh lesions compression should
   include the knee to avoid gravitational swelling into the joint
3. Elevation
4. Isometric exercises
5. Circulatory exercises to limb
6. Ultrasound
7. Short wave diathermy. Indirect application for wider circulatory
   problems
   Directly given to site only after haematoma is more isolated
8. Progressive exercises within pain limit

9. Gentle stretching after the inflammatory reaction has subsided
10. Modified massage at later stages

Complication
Myositis ossificans

Bursitis
Bursitis is included in this section because injuries affecting the deeper bursae are usually part of a more complicated disturbance already mentioned. The more isolated types of bursitis are those which are obvious because of their superficial position.

Cause
A direct heavy blow
Repeated less severe blows
Continual pressure
Prepatellar and olecranon bursitis are common particularly in body contact sports and in miners

Signs and symptoms
1. Swelling usually localized
2. Pain on pressure
3. Pain on any movement which increases pressure on the walls of the envelope of membrane

Principles of physiotherapy
Dispersion of the fluid whilst maintaining normal range is important as the initial inflammatory reaction subsides.

Possible techniques
1. Cold therapy if seen at time of injury
2. Rest and support
3. Ultrasound
4. Localized short wave diathermy
5. Progressive exercise within limit of pain and which does not put pressure on the bursa
6. Chronic stage. Massage including marginal frictions
7. Surgical removal may be necessary

This brief outline includes only some techniques particularly in the later stages. First aid measures for all soft tissue injuries should include:
1. Application of cold
   The exception to this is external bleeding, which must be controlled before any further treatment
2. Compression to provide support
The most important factor is the use of exercise. Electrotherapy may help. The co-operation of all concerned is essential but not always easy to achieve, especially in sport.

FURTHER READING

Adams, I. D. (1972) The management of the injured sportsman. *Physiotherapy*, **58**, 6–200.

Adams, J. C. (1986) *Outline of Orthopaedics*. 10th edition. Edinburgh: Churchill Livingstone.

Downie, P. A. (1984) *Textbook of General Medical and Surgical Conditions for Physiotherapists*. London: Faber & Faber.

Ellis, M. (1972) *Casualty Officers Handbook*. London: Butterworth.

Gordon, H. M. (1975) Physiotherapy in muscle strains of the lower limb. *Physiotherapy*, **61**, 4, 102.

O'Donaghue, D. H. (1950) The surgical treatment of fresh injuries to the major ligaments of the knee. *Journal of Bone and Joint Surgery*, **32A**, 721.

Steele, V. (1976) St. James' Hospital Sports Clinic. *Physiotherapy*, **62**, 8, 246.

Wiles, P. & Sweetman, R. (1965) *Essentials of Orthopaedics*. London: Churchill.

12. Diseases of joints

CLASSIFICATION

Group A: arthritis of unknown cause
Group B: arthritis due to infection
Group C: degenerative joint disease
Group D: crystal arthritis
Group E: connective tissue diseases

GROUP A – ARTHRITIS OF UNKNOWN CAUSE

Rheumatoid arthritis
Chronic systemic disease. Ranges from few joints mildly affected to complete ankylosis, and bed-ridden state. Age of onset puberty to old age. Two thirds before age 50. M1 : F3.

Signs and symptoms
1. Polyarthritis, often symmetrical
2. Small joints in hands and feet affected first (particularly 2nd and 3rd metacarpo-phalangeal and proximal interphalangeal joints)
3. Pain on movement
4. Morning stiffness of variable duration
5. Synovial thickening
6. Joints inflamed, painful and tender
7. Loss of range of movement
8. Flexion contractures
9. Finger deformities
    (i) Swan neck
    (ii) Ulnar deviation
    (iii) Boutonnière
    (iv) Subluxation
10. Clawed toes and callosities under MT heads
11. Valgus ankles
12. Generally valgus knees
13. Rheumatoid nodules on extensor surfaces
14. Thin skin
15. General malaise

Radiographic features
1. Soft tissue swellings
2. Osteoporosis
3. Loss of joint space
4. Bone erosions
5. Subluxation and deformity
6. Bony ankylosis

Pathological changes
1. Joints
    (i) Synovial inflammation and proliferation
    (ii) Synovial thickening and engorgement
    (iii) Cartilage erosions – pannus
    (iv) Cyst formation in bone
    (v) Bone loss
    (vi) Inflammation of synovial tendon sheaths
    (vii) Erosion and rupture of tendons
    (viii) Large synovial cysts
2. Vascular changes
    (i) Small arteries occluded – vasculitis
    (ii) Ulcers
    (iii) Neuropathies sensory and motor
3. Nerve entrapment
    (i) At carpal tunnel
    (ii) Behind elbow
    (iii) Round fibula head
4. Chest
    (i) Nodules in lung
    (ii) Pleural effusions
    (iii) Interstitial fibrosis
5. Eye
    (i) Inflammatory changes
    (ii) Dry eyes (Sjögren's syndrome)
    (iii) Sight impairment
6. General
    (i) Nodule formation
    (ii) Anaemia
    (iii) Elevated erythrocyte sedimentation rate or plasma viscosity level
    (iv) Positive rheumatoid factor tests in 80% cases
    (v) Atlanto-axial subluxation
    (vi) Amyloidosis
    (vii) Renal involvement
    (viii) Skin thinning
    (ix) Weight loss
    (x) Osteoporosis

Assessment
Observe:
1. General appearance
2. Gait
3. Deformity
4. Attitude to disease and condition
Enquire:
1. Actual age
2. Duration and severity of present illness
3. Sites of pain
4. Special difficulties
5. Home circumstances
6. Work circumstances
7. Family commitments
8. People/services already assisting
9. Drug therapy
10. Past medical history
Examination:
1. All joints for heat, tenderness and swelling, crepitus, laxity, deformity
2. Range of all movements
3. Assess motor power
Assess:
1. Likely response to treatment
2. Help required from other agencies
3. OT
   Social worker
   DRO

Principles of management
General:
1. Drug therapy must be adequate
2. Working against pain does not increase muscle power
3. Over-exertion should be avoided
Acute stage – pain relief:
1. Anti-inflammatory and analgesic drugs (NSAID)
2. Bed rest for acutely painful joints
3. Use splints if necessary
4. Ice packs for pain relief
5. Maintain ROM (Act. Ass. Movt.)
Subacute – increase mobility:
1. Ice packs
2. Gentle active movements
3. Isometric contractions
4. Hydrotherapy
5. Weight bearing after muscle control is achieved
6. Avoid sticks, crutches etc., to preserve upper limb joints

Chronic stage:
1. Encourage mobility
2. Increase muscle power
3. Give necessary walking aids: Fischer sticks, gutter, rotator, forearm crutches
4. Advise on self care

Treatment methods
Pain relief:
1. Rest
2. Ice packs or 2 lb bags of frozen peas. Latter are reusable
3. Wax e.g. for hands
4. Heat but not for inflamed joints
5. Resting splints. Plaster of Paris or plastazote
6. Relaxation – general and hydrotherapy
Mobilizing:
1. Exercises within pain-free range
2. Particular attention to neck and shoulder girdle
3. Suspension exercises
4. Spring assisted or lightly resisted exercise
5. Pendular exercises
6. Hydrotherapy
Strengthening:
1. Graduated isometric exercise
2. Introduce isotonic exercise
3. Pay particular attention to postural muscles
4. Hydrotherapy – graduated exercises against buoyancy
Advice:
1. Adequate rest periods
2. Housework programme
3. Home exercise programme
4. Keep weight down
5. If necessary
  (i) Alter furniture
  (ii) Provide handrails
  (iii) Provide walking aids and splints to protect joints
  (iv) Change employment
After initial treatment re-assess:
1. Residual disability
2. Patient's disposition
3. Attitude to disease
4. Relationship with family and workmates
5. Ability and desire to respond to treatment
6. Advisability of further therapy

Surgical treatment
In suitable cases a programme may include:
1. Synovectomy, tendon grafts/repair, removal of nodules

2. Excision arthroplasty
3. Interposition arthroplasty
4. Partial or total joint replacement
5. Arthrodesis

Where operative treatment not indicated
Appropriate aids may include:
1. Supportive splints
    (i) Wrists: Orthoplast polythene or Futuro
    (ii) Knees: Glassona, polythene or metal caliper or telescopic valgus support
    (iii) Ankles: Polythene or metal caliper
2. Walking aids: Sticks, crutches, light pick-ups
3. Special shoes of soft leather incorporating
    (i) Insoles
    (ii) Heel flares
    (iii) Raises or wedges
4. Wheelchairs: indoor/outdoor/electric

Juvenile rheumatoid arthritis
Several types:
One or two large joints affected
Polyarthritis similar to adults
Polyarthritis with systemic illness
Polyarthritis leading to ankylosing spondylitis
Peak age of onset 2–4 years
Second peak before puberty
Only 5% carry diseases to adulthood

Signs and symptoms
1. Joint inflammation
2. Onset in larger joints
3. Spinal involvement
4. Tendency to ankylosis
5. Eye inflammation
6. Rheumatoid factor test usually negative

Principles of management
1. Relieve pain
2. Prevent deformity
3. Maintain mobility
4. Prolonged immobilization inadvisable
5. Education must be kept up

Treatment methods
See page 180.

Ankylosing spondylitis
Inflammatory arthritis of spine
Sexes affected equally
Males more severely
Onset 16–40 years

Signs and symptoms
1. Lumbar backache
2. Pain and stiffness after rest and early morning
3. Sacro-iliac joints tender to forced movement
4. Stiff back – progressive rigidity
5. Loss of lumbar curve
6. Progressive thoracic kyphosis
7. Forward extended head
8. Reduced chest expansion
9. Sunken chest and pot belly
10. Flexion contractures of hips and shoulders
11. Plantar fasciitis
12. Achilles tendonitis

Radiographic features
1. Sacro-iliac erosion and later fusion
2. Arthritic changes in apophyseal joints
3. Ligamentous ossification in spine
4. Squaring of vertebral bodies
5. New bone growth between vertebrae ('syndesmophytes')
6. Peripheral joint erosions

Pathological changes
1. Ligamentous and capsular inflammation
2. Synovial inflammation
3. Ossification
4. Ankylosis
5. Rheumatoid factor tests negative
6. ESR raised
7. Tissue type HLA B27 positive in 90%

Complications
1. Reduced chest expansion and vital capacity
2. Possibility of chest infection
3. Atlanto-axial subluxation
4. Possible cord damage
5. Fractures of rigid spine
6. 10% cases have iritis
7. Associated ulcerative bowel disease
8. Amyloidosis
9. Heart disease

Assessment
Measure:
1. Chest expansion below nipple line
2. Occiput-wall distance, standing with heels to wall
3. Schroeber's index, i.e. mark 4/5 lumbar space, mark 10 cm upwards. Measure between marks on forward flexion
4. Vital capacity
5. Range of other joint movement – peripheral
6. Height
7. ROM spine

Principles of management
1. Maintain and increase spinal mobility
2. Prevent and correct deformity
3. Increase chest expansion and vital capacity
4. Attention to posture
5. Drug therapy for relief of pain and stiffness
6. Advice to patient and self-help (National Ankylosing Spondylitis Society)

Treatment methods
Pain relief:
1. Analgesics and anti-inflammatory drugs
2. Heat
3. Hydrotherapy
Mobilizing:
1. Vigorous exercises including
   (i) Side flexion
   (ii) Rotation
   (iii) Extension of all parts of the spine
2. Hydrotherapy
3. Breathing exercises
4. Chest mobility exercises
5. Hip and shoulder exercises
6. Shoulder girdle exercises
7. Passive stretching to peripheral joints
Strengthening:
1. Back extension exercises
2. Postural exercises
Give short course of supervised treatment
Teach home exercises
Re-assess in 1 month
Treat if necessary
Thereafter re-assess yearly
Encourage and maintain long-term support service

Advice to patients
1. Education concerning the nature of the disease
2. Emphasize importance of daily exercise
3. Put a board under mattress
4. Use one pillow or none
5. Spend some time prone lying daily
6. Supine lying if prone impossible
7. Perform home exercises twice daily
8. Always be conscious of posture
9. Encourage a sport e.g. swimming

Adjust if necessary:
Height of work bench or desk
Chair
Teach best method of performing daily tasks
Driving mirrors and seat height

Reiter's disease
A combination of urethritis and arthritis
Attacks young men
Usually develops from sexually transmitted non-specific urethritis
May follow dysentry
The venereal type rare in women

Signs and symptoms
1. Urethral discharge: dysuria
2. Acute arthritis follows in 10–21 days
3. Arthritis commonly affects knees, ankles and feet
4. Other peripheral joints may be affected
5. Systemic reaction
6. Fever
7. Weight loss
8. General malaise
9. Conjunctivitis with sterile eye discharge (40%)
10. Mouth and genital ulceration (10%)
11. Keratoderma blennorrhagica on hands and feet (10%)

Radiographic features
Similar to rheumatoid arthritis

Pathological changes
1. Urethritis
2. Synovial proliferation and effusion
3. Tendonitis around ankle
4. Plantar fasciitis
5. Erosive arthritis
6. Genital and mouth ulceration
7. Reiter's cells (large macrophages) in synovial fliud

Principles of management
1. Treat venereal disease
2. Acute arthritic symptoms treated as for rheumatoid arthritis
3. Surgery may become necessary in persistent or recurrent cases
4. Advice about re-infection and disease recurrence

Treatment methods
1. Oxy-tetracyline for urethritis
2. Anti-inflammatory drugs
3. Joint aspiration
4. Intra-articular injection of steroids
5. Bed rest with splints if necessary
6. Ice packs
7. Graduated active exercises, especially quadriceps
8. Weight bearing when good muscle control is established

Psoriatic arthropathy
Psoriasis. May be small skin or scalp patches
Nail pitting and ridging
Little systemic upset
Rheumatoid factor tests negative
Varied joint disease:
1. Erosive terminal joint disease in hands and feet
2. Polyarthritis but less symmetrical than rheumatoid arthritis.
   Flexor tendon involvement, spindle swelling/sausage digit
3. Sacro-iliac and spinal arthritis
4. Rare, destructive arthritis mutilans in hands and feet, opera
   glass digits
Treatment as for rheumatoid arthritis.

GROUP B – ARTHRITIS DUE TO INFECTION

Rheumatic fever
A disease of decreasing incidence and severity
Affects young people

Signs and symptoms
1. Fever
2. Infection of the throat
3. Skin rash
4. Transient polyarthritis
5. Subcutaneous nodules
6. General malaise

Pathological changes
1. Streptococcal infection
2. Inflammatory synovitis of joints

3. Inflammatory damage to the heart
4. Cardiac arrhythmias
5. Mitral or aortic valve disease
6. Possible permanent heart damage
7. Produces disability at times of cardiac strain e.g. pregnancy

Principles of management
1. Drug therapy
2. Bed rest
3. No need for splints
4. Progressive mobilization

Treatment methods
Acute stage:
1. Antibiotics for streptococcal infection
2. Analgesic and anti-inflammatory drugs
3. Bed rest
4. Ice packs
5. Gentle active movements
Subacute stage:
1. Progressive mobilization
2. Graduated active exercise
3. Palliative ice or heat
4. Suspension exercises
5. Hydrotherapy
Chronic stage:
1. Prophylactic long-term antibiotics
2. Assessment of cardiac damage
3. Advice about activity levels

Septic arthritis
Bacterial infection of joint introduced by operation, trauma or injection
May spread from infection elsewhere
Metal prostheses may attract bacteria

Signs and symptoms
1. Any joint may be affected, usually monoarticular
2. Acutely painful
3. Inflamed
4. Fever
5. Raised erythrocyte sedimentation rate
6. Commonly, staphylococcal infection

Principles of management
1. Identify source of infection
2. Bacteriological culture of synovial fluid and blood
3. Suitable antibiotics
4. Surgical drainage if necessary

5. Rest, often with splints
6. Later mobilization

Arthritis may also occur in association with other infections:
1. Gonorrhoea
2. Brucellosis
3. Tuberculosis
4. Erythema nodosum
5. Some virus diseases
6. Ulcerative colitis

GROUP C – DEGENERATIVE JOINT DISEASE

Monoarticular osteoarthrosis or secondary osteoarthritis

Predisposing factors
1. Development e.g. Perthes'
2. Inflammatory e.g. RA, AS
3. Infective arthritis
4. Metabolic e.g. Paget's
5. Previous trauma
6. Abnormal weight distribution e.g. poliomyelitis
7. Occupation
8. Endocrine factors

Signs and symptoms
1. Hip and knee joints most commonly attacked
2. Pain on movement
3. Pain – rest/night
        – referred
4. Muscle spasm
5. Progressive loss of range of movement
6. Joint stiffness after rest
7. Moderate effusion
8. Bony swelling and osteophyte formation
9. Crepitus; sometimes audible
10. Hip deformity, usually
    (i) Adduction
    (ii) Flexion
    (iii) Lateral rotation
11. Knee deformity usually
    (i) Varus/valgus
    (ii) Flexion
12. Leg length discrepancy due to fixed flexion

Radiographic features
1. Diminished joint space
2. Sclerosis of subchrondral bone
3. Cysts in subchondral bone
4. New bone growth: osteophytes

5. Loose bodies
6. Subluxation of joint and deformity

Pathological changes
1. Fibrillation of articular cartilage
2. Thinning of articular cartilage
3. Subchondral bone sclerosis
4. Osteophyte formation
5. Eburnation
6. Calcification of cartilage – loose bodies
7. Cyst formation in bone
8. Collapse of joint surfaces
9. Subluxation of joint
10. Bony ankylosis

Precipitating pathology may be
1. Obesity
2. Congenital abnormalities
3. Perthes' disease and related bone damage in adolescents
4. Rheumatoid or other arthritis
5. Trauma
6. Fracture

Assessment
Observe:
1. General appearance and posture
2. Gait
3. If stick or walking aid used
4. If overweight or obese
Enquire:
1. Site and duration of pain
2. If night pain
3. If precipitated by other pathology
4. Special difficulties
5. Nature of employment
Examine hip joint:
1. Measure range of movement
    (i) Active
    (ii) Passive
2. Measure leg lengths for
    (i) True
    (ii) Apparent shortening
3. Palpate for
    (i) Tender areas
    (ii) Muscle spasm
4. Assess power of all muscle groups
5. Carry out Trendelenburg test

Examine other joints:
1. Observe redness and swelling
2. Palpate for
    (i) Heat
    (ii) Tenderness
    (iii) Muscle spasm
3. Measure joint circumference
4. Measure range of movement
    (i) Active
    (ii) Passive
5. Assess muscle power
6. Compare with contralateral joint

Principles of management
1. Pain relief
2. Increase mobility
3. Increase muscle power
4. Advice on self-help/independence
5. Surgical treatment

Treatment methods
To reduce pain and muscle spasm:
1. Drug therapy
2. Ice packs
3. Short wave diathermy
    Caution. Heat treatment may aggravate symptoms
4. Ultrasound/interferential
5. Hydrotherapy
6. Suspension exercises
7. Traction with care!
To mobilize:
1. Passive mobilizations 'Maitlands'
2. Positioning of patient e.g. prone lying
3. Pulley exercises
4. Traction
5. Suspension exercises
6. Active movements
7. Hydrotherapy
8. PNF – hold/relax
9. Pendular exercises
10. Traction with care!
To increase muscle power:
1. Proprioceptive neuromuscular facilitation techniques
2. Isometric and isotonic exercises
3. Pulley exercises
4. Graduated resisted exercises
5. Hydrotherapy

To improve function:
1. Postural exercises
2. Gait training
3. Supply if required
   (i) Walking aids
   (ii) Splints made of: Plastazote
                        Plaster of Paris
                        Glassona
                        Polythene
                        T.V.'s
   (iii) Footwear incorporating: Insoles
                                Heel flares
                                Heel cups
                                Wedges

Surgical treatment
1. Osteotomy
2. Excision arthroplasty
3. Interposition arthroplasty
4. Partial or total joint replacement
5. Arthrodesis
For postoperative management see orthopaedic section.

Advice to patient
1. Diet and weight control
2. Home exercises
3. Use of walking aids
4. Use of household aids
5. Adaptation of furniture
Re-assess patient and review treatment at intervals.

Generalized osteoarthrosis or primary osteoarthritis
Attacks the middle aged to elderly
Women more than men particularly postmenopausal. F10:M1
Strong genetic influence

Signs and symptoms
1. Characteristic bony swellings on terminal phalanges (Heberden nodes) and proximal phalanges (Bouchard's nodes)
2. Painful polyarthritis
3. Joints become tender and thickened
4. May be inflamed
5. Joint stiffness
6. Painful joints
7. Progressive loss of range of movement
8. Fine crepitus
9. Deformity

Joints most commonly affected:
1. Distal inter-phalangeal of hands
2. First carpometacarpal
3. Other joints of hand
4. Knee

Radiographic and pathological changes as in monoarticular osteoarthrosis.

Assessment
As for monoarticular disease.

Principles of management
As for monoarticular disease
Surgery is less frequently indicated except for 1st carpometacarpal joint.

Cervico-lumbar spondylosis and disc degeneration
Affects adults past middle age
Depression is often a feature

Cervical spine: signs and symptoms
Apophyseal joints:
1. Neck pain. Aggravated by movement
2. Stiffness
3. Limitation of movement
4. Crepitus

Intervertebral discs:
Commonly C5–7 level
1. Aching pain
2. Increasing to severe pain
3. Limitation of movement

Nerve root compression:
1. Radiating pain
2. Paraesthesia
3. Decreased reflexes in root distribution
4. Muscle weakness

Cord compression:
Common level C5–6
Increased leg reflexes
Sensory abnormalities in arms and legs

Vertebral artery compression:
Movement precipitates –
1. Visual disturbances
2. Transient blackouts

Lumbar spine: signs and symptoms
Apophyseal joints – less frequently affected:
1. Pain aggravated by movement
2. Rigid back
3. Limited movements
Intervertebral discs – usually L 4–5 or L 5–S1 level:
1. Low back pain
2. Aggravated by coughing or sneezing
3. Sciatic pain increased by nerve stretching
4. Muscle spasm
5. Scoliosis
6. Loss of lumbar curve
7. Flexion limited
Nerve root compression:
1. Radiating pain
2. Paraesthesia
3. Numbness
4. Diminished or absent reflexes
5. Muscle weakness
Cauda equina compression:
1. Back pain
2. Bilateral radiating pain
3. Bilateral paralysis
4. Bilateral sensory loss
5. Loss of sphincter control

Acute disc lesions
Usually traumatic in origin
Affect a younger more active age group

Signs and symptoms
1. Sudden acute onset
2. Severe pain
3. Spasm
4. Scoliosis
5. Loss of spinal movement

Nerve root and cord compression symptoms
As described above but more acute.

Radiographic features
X-ray changes do not necessarily correlate with symptoms,
especially in cervical region.
1. Reduced joint spaces
2. Reduced disc spaces
3. Arthritic changes in apophyseal joints
4. Bone sclerosis
5. Alteration of normal spinal curves
6. Scoliosis

7. Osteophyte formation
8. Myelogram may show disc protrusion and nerve root compression

Pathological changes
Degenerative disease:
1. Osteoarthrotic changes in joints
2. Degenerative changes in annulus fibrosus
3. Extrusion of nucleus pulposus
4. Bone cyst formation
5. Osteophyte formation
6. Kinking of vertebral arteries
Traumatic disease:
1. Tear of vertebral muscles
2. Tear of interspinal ligaments
3. Apophyseal joint subluxation
4. Disc prolapse

Assessment
1. Medical and radiographic investigations must first be carried out
2. Obtain accurate history
3. Examination
    (i) Presence of spasm and scoliosis
    (ii) Palpate for tenderness
    (iii) Range of movement in all planes
    (iv) Effect of movement
        a. Active
        b. Passive
    (v) Appropriate nerve stretch tests
    (iv) Test sensation

Principles of management
1. Pain relief
    (i) Analgesics
    (ii) Rest
    (iii) Heat
    (iv) Traction
    (v) Passive manipulation
2. Spinal support
    (i) Plaster jacket or corset
    (ii) Cervical collar
3. Postural re-education
4. Advise patient on self-care
5. Surgical intervention
    To decompress nerve roots or cord:
    (i) Laminectomy
    (ii) Discectomy
    (iii) Spinal fusion

Treatment methods

Acute stages:
1. Analgesics
2. Bed rest. Possibly prolonged
3. Heat packs
4. Head traction for cervical lesions
5. Pelvic or leg traction for lumbar lesions
6. Mobilizations

Subacute stage:
1. Local heat. Infrared. Short wave diathermy
2. Passive mobilizations
3. Active movements progressed gently
4. Exercises:
   Neck
   Shoulder girdle
   Abdomen
   Leg extension
5. Support if required
   (i) Cervical collar appropriately firm
   (ii) Corset or plaster jacket
6. Check gait and posture

Recovery stage:
1. Work towards full mobility
2. Progressively vigorous exercises for
   (i) Spine; all sections
   (ii) Shoulder girdle
   (iii) Abdominal wall
   (iv) Pelvic girdle
   (v) Legs
3. Gait and posture
4. Advice
   (i) Simple regime of home exercises
   (ii) Board under mattress
   (iii) Lifting techniques
   (iv) Avoidance of strain
   (v) Suitable sport and activity
   (vi) Suitable chair at home and work
   (vii) Adaptation of work situation

GROUP D – CRYSTAL ARTHRITIS

Gout

Affects adult males
Women after menopause

Signs and symptoms
1. Severe pain cf. septic arthritis
2. Local inflammation
3. Any joint. Usually monoarticular
4. Commonest in 1st MTP joint
5. Uncommon in hip or shoulder

Pathological changes
1. In joint
    (i) Inflammatory
    (ii) Often violent reaction
    (iii) Uric acid crystals in synovial fluid
2. Systemic
    (i) Raised plasma uric acid
    (ii) Raised white cell count
    (iii) Raised ESR
3. Complications
    (i) Tophi, urate deposits in soft tissues
    (ii) Secondary degenerative arthritis
    (iii) Renal disease

Medical treatment
Drug therapy:
1. Indomethacin, Phenylbutazone for acute attack
2. Allopurinol for long-term prevention
Physiotherapy not usually indicated.

Pseudo-gout

Affects either sex
Usually over 45 years

Signs and symptoms
1. Usually monoarticular
2. Commonly knee, shoulder or wrist
3. Joint hot, tender, swollen and painful
4. Synovial effusion
5. Occasionally insidious and polyarticular cf. rheumatoid arthritis
6. Occasionally insidious and cause of osteoarthrosis

Medical treatment
1. Analgesic and anti-inflammatory drugs
2. Joint aspiration
3. Intra-articular corticosteroid injections

Physiotherapy treatment
1. Ice packs
2. Early mobilization
3. Restoration of muscle strength and bulk
4. Weight bearing exercises

GROUP E – CONNECTIVE TISSUE DISEASES

Scleroderma
A rare progressive disease of unknown cause

Signs and symptoms
1. Raynaud's phenomenon
2. Tight shiny skin
3. Sclerodactyly
4. Telangiectasia
5. Calcinosis
6. Slightly swollen joints
7. Loss of range of movement
8. Skin ulceration
9. Oesophageal stricture

Pathological changes
1. Increased collagen production
2. Skin tethering
3. Fibrosis of lungs, kidneys and intestines
4. Mild synovitis

Complications
1. Hypertension
2. Malnutrition
3. Heart and lung failure

Principles of management
1. Treat complications
2. Encourage mobility
3. Drugs of doubtful value

Treatment methods (see p. 147)
1. Drug therapy
2. Wax for hands and feet
3. Gentle passive stretching
4. Active movements
5. Ulcer care including ultraviolet light

Advice to patient
1. Keep extremities warm
2. Regular daily exercise

Other connective tissue diseases
1. Dermatomyositis
2. Disseminated lupus erythematosis
3. Polymyalgia rheumatica
4. Polyarteritis nodosa

Polymyalgia rheumatica
Patients over 55 years
Women more frequently

Signs and symptoms
1. Shoulder-girdle pain
2. Sometimes pelvic pain
3. Severe morning stiffness in girdles
4. Tenderness in musculature, no wasting
5. General ill health

Complications
Temporal arteritis and blindness

Treatment
Corticosteroid therapy – dramatic effect

Physiotherapy management
Treatment is symptomatic
Advice on rest activity cycle

FURTHER READING

Boyle, J. & Buchanan, W. W. (1971) *Clinical Rheumatology*. Oxford: Blackwell.

Day, B. H. (1972) *Orthopaedic Appliances*. London: Faber & Faber

Downie, P. A. (1984) *Textbook of Orthopaedics and Rheumatology for Physiotherapist's*. London: Faber & Faber.

Goble, R. E. A. & Nicholls, P. J. R. (1971) *Rehabilitation of Severely Disabled*. Vols 1 and 2. London: Butterworth.

Haslock, I. & Wright, V. (1977) *Rheumatism for Nurses and Remedial Therapists*. London: Heinemann.

Hollander, J. L. & McCarthy, D. J. eds. (1972) *Arthritis and Allied Conditions. A Textbook of Rheumatology*. Philadelphia: Lea & Febiger.

Mason, M. & Currey, H. L. F. eds. (1970) *An Introduction to Clinical Rheumatology*. London: Pitman.

Scott, J. T. ed. (1977) *Textbook of Rheumatic Diseases*. Edinburgh: Churchill Livingstone.

13. Paediatric conditions

Paediatric physiotherapy is the Politics of the Possible. Physiotherapy is but one aspect of a child's life; it must never become an end in itself but remain one of the means of enabling a child to lead as independent and full a life as possible. The paediatric physiotherapist is very much a small cog in the very big wheel of team effort. The participation and co-operation of the child's family is essential.

CEREBRAL PALSY

A permanent disorder of movement and posture with sensory defects, due to brain damage or developmental abnormality occurring in fetal life or early infancy. Progression of clinical features due to child's developmental progress.

Causes
1. Birth injury
2. Anoxia
3. Prematurity
4. Intracranial infections
5. Trauma

Types
1. *Spastic quadriplegia*
   (i) Hypertonus of whole body even at rest
   (ii) Primitive responses present
   (iii) Rigidity
   (iv) Contractures and deformities may be present
   (v) Head control poor
   (vi) Often impairment of speech and sight
   (vii) Asymmetry of posture and movement
2. *Spastic diplegia*
   (i) Delayed milestones
   (ii) Whole body affected, legs more than arms
   (iii) Good head control
   (iv) Increasingly obvious spastic patterns of movement

3. *Hemiplegia*
    (i) One side of body affected
    (ii) Asymmetry of posture and movement
    (iii) Balance reactions poor
    (iv) Parachute reactions diminished
    (v) Difference in growth and consequently length of the affected side

4. *Athetoid quadriplegia*
    (i) Often floppy in neonatal
    (ii) Increasing fluctuations in muscular tone
    (iii) Involuntary movements
    (iv) Little co-contraction of muscle groups
    (v) Hypermobility of joints
    (vi) Extreme dystonia fixed deformities may occur
    (vii) Abnormalities of breathing and speech

5. *Ataxia*
    (i) Cerebellar lesions
    (ii) Gross motor inco-ordination
    (iii) Poor, diminished balance and equilibrium reactions
    (iv) Intention tremor
    (v) High stepping gait
    (vi) Hypotonia

Principles of management
There are great similarities and overlap of symptoms and often it is difficult to differentiate the type of cerebral palsy. Therefore, treat according to problems presenting.

1. *Development assessment to determine*
    (i) Patterns of spasticity and tonic reflexes e.g. ATNR, TNR
    (ii) Abnormal associated reactions
    (iii) Primitive responses
    (iv) Balance and equilibrium reactions
    (v) Fluctuations in tone
    (vi) Contractures, muscle imbalance
    (vii) Symmetry. Asymmetry of posture, movement, growth
    (viii) Voluntary control
    (ix) Problems of perception, proprioception, spatial awareness, comprehension, communication etc.
    By placing the child, or asking the child to attain the following positions:
      a. Supine lying
      b. Prone lying
      c. Rolling
      d. Creeping
      e. Crawling
      f. Long-sitting
      g. Cross-legged sitting
      h. Half-kneeling

   i. High kneeling
   j. Prone kneeling
   k. Standing
   l. Walking

2. *Inhibit abnormal reflex activity*
 (i) Positioning
 (ii) Key points
 (iii) Reflex inhibiting movement patterns in sitting, lying, using roll or ball
 (iv) Shaking, rolling, tapping, compressions
 (v) Rebound therapy
 (vi) Yoga relaxation
 (vii) Hippotherapy

3. *Facilitate normal patterns of body movement*
 (i) Weight bearing in key positions
 (ii) Weight transference in key positions
 (iii) Shaking, rolling, tapping, compressions for balance control
 (iv) Rebound therapy
 (v) PNF
 (vi) Hippotherapy

4. *Stimulation of body awareness, perception, proprioception etc.*
 (i) Mirror work in key positions using roll, ball etc.
 (ii) Weight bearing and transference
 (iii) Yoga regime
 (iv) Rebound therapy
 Use any relevant technique as before.

5. *Contractures, deformities arising, prevention*
 e.g. Wind – sweeping; scoliosis; different limb length; fixed pelvic tilt
 (i) Correct functional seating and standing using standing frames, moulded inserts, adapted chairs, prone boards, side lying boards etc.
 (ii) Splinting – dynamic or resting
  a. Serial splinting
  b. Night splinting
  c. Abduction splinting
  d. DFO
  e. Alterations to footwear e.g. Piedro boots, crooked and elongated heels etc.
 (iii) Surgery
  a. Closed tenotomies
  b. Open tenotomies
  c. Tendon transplants e.g. Eggers' operation

6. *Constant correction and re-education of posture*

PERTHES' DISEASE (PSEUDOCOXALGIA)

Cause
Unknown; possibilities, excessive strain on growing bone;
generalized skeletal developmental disorder; hypothyroidism.

Pathological changes
Avascular necrosis of the femoral head (occasionally bilateral) with
cystic cavities being gradually filled with new bone. Can result in
residual deformity of the femoral head. Most common in boys 4–10
years old.

Clinical features
1. Limp with or without pain
2. On X-ray, increase density, followed by fragmentation and re-
ossification
3. Limitation of abduction and internal rotation

Management
Depends entirely on orthopaedic consultant's regime.
1. Intermittent short-term immobilization when pain present,
interspersed with free active exercises to maintain mobility
2. Long-term immobilization can be up to 2 years in frog-leg
plasters
3. Non-weight bearing full leg caliper
Physiotherapists follow individual consultant's regime but the
following techniques apply:
(i) Hydrotherapy
(ii) Back extension, glutei strengthening
(iii) Intensive re-education of walking

SPINA BIFIDA

Cause
Unknown

Pathological changes
Congenital abnormality with developmental defect of spinal
column with incomplete closure of the vertebral canal.

Spina bifida cystica
As above, with protrusion and dysplasia of spinal cord and
membranes forming a meningocele or myelomeningocele.
Problems occurring according to site of the lesion.

Clinical features
1. Flaccid paralysis
2. Muscle weakness
3. Decrease or absent tendon reflexes

4. Impaired proprioception and sensation
5. Incontinence
6. Congenital deformities, feet, hips, spine
7. Hydrocephalus

Spina bifida occulta
No herniation or displacement of meninges.
Neurological signs may or may not be present.

Management of neonatal problems
1. *Myelomeningocele*
   Surgery at parents/consultant's discretion
2. *Hydrocephalus*
   Insertion of drainage valve – Spitz-Holter valve
   Complications:
   (i) Infection at site of valve
   (ii) Blockage of valve
   Both these may result in loss, impaired vision, impaired intellect
   (iii) Weight of enlarged head influences head control.
   Positioning of head in lying very important
3. *Talipes equino-varus*
   (i) Splintage or strapping – remembering impaired sensation
   (ii) Passive movements
4. *Dislocation of hips*
   (i) Splintage – remember impaired sensation
   (ii) Passive movements
   (iii) Positioning in cot

Long-term management
Active participation of parents essential.
1. Developmental assessment and muscle power chart
2. Encourage normal developmental progression
   (i) Head control
   (ii) Rolling
   (iii) Sitting from lying
   (iv) Creeping etc.
   (v) Standing by year using orthopaedic standing frames i.e.
   Orlau or Shrewsbury; pelvic band calipers etc.
   (vi) Balance and equilibrium reactions in sitting and standing
   (vii) Develop spatial awareness, perception, body image
   (viii) Maintain joint range to minimize contractures
   (ix) Strengthen extensor muscles
   (x) Strengthen upper arms and thorax
   (xi) Mobility using wheelchairs, walking aids
   (xii) Functional independence in transferring wheelchair
   mobility; dressing; putting on calipers; outdoor
   wheelchair mobility; toilet; skin care
   (xiii) Breathing exercise to increase chest expansion

CYSTIC FIBROSIS (MUCOVISCIDOSIS)

Cause
Unknown.
Recessive autosomal gene.

Pathological changes
A disturbance of the exocrine glands, resulting in increased production of viscid mucus.

Clinical features
1. Intestinal obstruction in neonatal resulting in meconium ileus
2. Malabsorption due to pancreatic insufficiency results in failure to thrive, poor weight gain, diarrhoea, offensive stools, rectal collapse
3. Recurrent respiratory infections, progressive bronchiectasis, emphysema, cor pulmonale
4. Excess secretion of salt in sweat

Management
1. Meconium ileus: surgery to remove blockage
2. Malabsorption, improved occasionally by low fat diet, added pancreatin
3. Respiratory problems – control of infection
   Key to survival:
      (i) Regular home visits to gain the co-operation and participation of family
      (ii) Teach postural drainage techniques as soon as possible
      (iii) Advise on necessary equipment to facilitate drainage techniques i.e. sag bags, wedges etc.
      (iv) Encourage activities to increase exercise tolerance i.e. Trampette, gymnastics, dancing etc.
      (v) Teach inhalation and nebulizer techniques if necessary
      (vi) Teach forced expiration techniques if the child is old enough to undertake own PD
      (vii) Postural correction exercises, thoracic mobility

FRIEDREICH'S ATAXIA

Cause
Unknown: autosomal recessive gene.

Pathological changes
1.. Progressive cerebellar and spinal cord dysfunction
2. Atrophy of cardiac muscles
3. Degeneration of spinocerebellar, posterior column and cortico spinal tracts

Clinical features
1. Cortico spinal tract dysfunction
   Positive Babinski
2. Peripheral neuropathy
   (i) Loss of tendon reflexes
   (ii) Distal weakness
   (iii) Muscle atrophy
3. Cerebellar dysfunction
   (i) Progressive ataxic gait
   (ii) Dysarthria
   (iii) Intention tremor
   (iv) Nystagmus
4. Development of scoliosis, pes cavus, hammer toes
5. Loss of independent ambulation
6. Eventual cardiomegaly, arrhythmia, cardiac failure

Management
1. No effective chemotherapy
2. Surgical intervention not advisable
3. Physiotherapy management
   (i) Treat according to symptoms presenting (see CP notes for Ataxia)
   (ii) Maintain joint range – passive stretching
   (iii) Posture re-education. Strengthen antigravity muscles
   (iv) Appropriate appliances i.e. weighted boots
   (v) Wheelchair
   (vi) Mouded insert may be useful to help prevent scoliosis
   (vii) Frenkel's exercises

ARTHROGYPHOSIS MULTIFLEX CONGENITA

Cause
Unknown.
Intra-uterine pressure.

Pathological changes
Frequent associated defects, i.e. sacral agenesis, cleft palate etc. presuppose origin in early fetal life.
1. Thick inelastic articular capsules
2. Atrophy, hypoplasia of muscle fibres
3. Fibrous and fatty refiltration of muscle fibres
4. Cartilaginous facial features
5. Degeneration of anterior horn cells of spinal cord

Clinical features
1. Congenital stiffness and deformity of one or more joints
2. Limb joints fused in either flexion or extension
3. Dislocation of joints (frequently hip joints)

4. Severe talipes, valgus deformities, hands
5. Lack major muscle groups i.e. gluteii, quads.

Physiotherapy management
Parental involvement straight away. Explain long-term prospect
and encourage often.
1. Neonatal
    (i) Surgery. Intensive splintage and stretching
    (ii) Encourage normal developmental sequence
2. Long-term plan
    (i) Maintain and improve joint range
    (ii) Developmental sequence
    (iii) Strengthen existing muscle groups
    (iv) Careful consideration and supervision of calipers etc.
    (v) Encourage functional independence
    (vi) Stimulate ambulation, select appropriate walking aid,
        wheelchair
    (vii) Hydrotherapy

Congenital dislocation of hip

Cause
Unknown.
1. Genetic factor. Familial lax joints, shallow acetabular rim?
2. Breech baby
3. Spina-bifida
4. Females – joint laxity caused by formation of relaxin in uterus

Pathological changes
Dislocation, dysplasia of femoral head, dysplasia of acetabulum,
lax ligaments.

Diagnosis
All babies are screened at birth.
Ortolani's sign: a palpable click felt on manipulation, with flexed
hip and knee abducted 90°

Management
1. Early TR – splintage, Dennis Brown harness 6–12 months. No
   future recurrence
2. After 12 months – open reduction
3. Established deformity
    (i) De-rotation osteotomy
    (ii) Salter osteotomy of pelvis
    (iii) Acetabuloplasty
4. Later life (often spina-bifida)
    (i) Arthrodesis
    (ii) Total hip replacement

Physiotherapy management
Most cases resolve themselves. No further occurrence.
1. Encourage parental involvement
2. Mother/baby play regime to mobilize after fixation
3. Encourage normal developmental sequence
4. Individual exercise regime

ATAXIA TELANGIECTASIA

Autosomal recessive gene.
25% recurrence risk with siblings.

Pathological changes
(Immunological dysfunction associated with progressive
degeneration of cerebellum.)

Clinical features
1. Neurological – begin in infancy
   (i) No positive Babinski sign
   (ii) Delayed milestones – slow to walk, ataxic
   (iii) Later childhood: dysarthria; nystagmus; intention tremor;
        choreoathetosis; diminished tendon reflexes
   (iv) Scoliosis
   (v) Loss of independent ambulation
2. Immunological deficiency
   (i) Recurrent sinusitis, ENT infections, pulmonary infections
   (ii) Tonsillar tissue dim or absent
   (iii) No palpable lymph nodes

Prognosis
Poor because of pulmonary infection. 2 decade terminal. Increase
tendency to lymphomas; brain tumours.

Management
1. Gammaglobulin injections
2. Maintain, improve balance reactions, etc. (See Ataxia in CP
   conditions)
3. Frequent PD to relieve chest infections
4. Nebulize
5. Maintain spinal posture, prevent deformities
6. Supervise adequate bracing
7. Advise wheelchair seating – moulded inserts
8. Frenkel's exercises

MYOSITIS AND DERMATOMYOSITIS

Cause
Unknown.

Pathological changes
Myositis – general inflammatory changes in skeletal muscles, subcutaneous tissues and skin.
Dermatomyositis – widespread, patchy, erythematous rash.

Clinical features of acute phase
1. Muscle tenderness and pain
2. General malaise, low grade fever
3. Proximal weakness in limbs
4. Gower's sign present

Prognosis
Poor. Fulminating cases terminal within weeks of onset.

Management
Acute phase:
1. Steroids
2. Contractures develop rapidly
3. Position in bed
4. Daily passive movements
5. Light weight splinting
Sub-acute phase:
1. Mobilize
2. Hydrotherapy
3. Active assisted movements. All joints
4. Wax
5. Daily passive movements

MUSCULAR DYSTROPHY

Cause
Unknown.
Heredofamilial genetic disorder.

Pathological changes
A progressive atrophy of muscles which swell, undergo hyaline changes being replaced by connective tissue and fat. Other abnormalities: defective peripheral vasomotor control; sinus tachycardia; myocardial fibrosis.

Types
1. Pseudohypertrophic muscular dystrophy (Duchenne)
    (i) X-linked recessive gene
    (ii) Primarily boys (increase serum creatine-kinase and aldolase)
    (iii) Female carriers (increased serum creatine-kinase)
    (iv) Symptoms insidious but rapid course i.e. pelvic girdle muscles primarily, symmetrical progression includes pectoral girdle, trunk muscles, distal muscles, cardiac muscle
    (v) Gower's sign
    (vi) Pseudohypertrophy especially calf
    (vii) Contractures of distal joints
    (viii) Gradual loss of independent ambulation
    (ix) Scoliosis, kyphosis
    (x) Respiratory problems. Diminished vital capacity
2. Facioscapulohumeral
    (i) Autosomal dominant gene
    (ii) Benign disease of late childhood or adult life
    (iii) Insidious slow weakness in facial and pectoral muscles
    (iv) Winging scapula
    (v) Mouth droop, eyelids cannot close, face becomes mask like
3. Limb girdle
    (i) Autosomal dominant or recessive gene
    (ii) Insidious but rapid onset
    (iii) Pre-adolescents
    (iv) Affects shoulder, pelvic girdle (mainly pelvic)
    (v) Variable clinical manifestations
    (vi) Loss of independent ambulation
4. Myotonic (Thomsen's disease)
    (i) Autosomal dominant gene
    (ii) Boys and girls early childhood
    (iii) Muscle stiffness resulting from myotonia
    (iv) Significant weakness especially dorsiflexors
    (v) Focal involvement proximal girdle muscles
    (vi) Occasionally: baldness, lenticular cataracts, testicular atrophy, emotional disturbance

Management
1. Submaximal exercises avoid exhaustion
2. Hydrotherapy
3. Breathing exercises playing wind instruments
4. Vigorous stretchings using wedges, rolls etc.
5. Intermittent compression
6. Maintain standing for part of day using
    (i) Dynamic leg braces
    (ii) Long leg calipers

(iii) Swivel walkers
(iv) Standing frames
in order to:
(v) Reduce chest infections
(vi) Facilitate kidney and bowel function
(vii) Maintain normal bone structure
(viii) Prevent contractures
(ix) Prevent constriction of abdominal cavity
7. Lightweight night and day splintage lower limbs
8. Wheelchair life inevitable – prevent scoliosis by
(i) Electric wheelchair with mid-line control
(ii) Wedge-shaped cushion
(iii) Side wedges
(iv) Hard base (plywood) underneath cushion
(v) Moulded insert to prevent pelvic shift
(vi) Lumbar corset with hyperextension at lumbar spine
(viii) Attention to foot plate height

TALIPES EQUINOVARUS

Causes
1. Genetic
2. Infection in utero
3. Intra-uterine pressure
4. Drugs
5. Congenital neuromuscular abnormalities

Pathological changes
Underdeveloped shortening of soft tissues in medial aspect of foot, resulting in adducted, inverted foot with plantar flexed ankle, pipe stem calf. Can be bilateral. Severe cases: bones small, distorted. Associated congenital handicapping conditions i.e. spina-bifida, muscular dystrophy.

Management
Emphasis on early treatment within first 12 h.
1. Manipulation
Teach parents. Always flex knee, hip before stretching. Adduct and invert foot and then correct equinus
2. Active exercises
Encourage parents to help exercise infant
3. Splintage
(i) POP knee 90°
(ii) Dennis Browne boots
(iii) Strapping. Tinct. benz. protect skin. Pad pressure points.
(iv) Night splints. Serial splints
4. Surgery 12 weeks → 6 months severe cases
(i) Soft tissue release A/K. POP knee flexion 90° 6–8 weeks

(ii) Calcaneal osteotomy A/K. POP 10° knee flexion 6–8 weeks. Usually for later diagnosis
(iii) Adolescence. Tendon transplant. Tibialis posterior
(iv) Growth complete. Triple arthrodesis

SCLERODERMA

Cause
Unknown.

Pathological changes
Similar to dermatomyositis.
The skin becomes thickened with deposit of collagen fibres.
Calcinosis may occur. Morphea bands may be present.

Prognosis
Childhood onset better chance of remission, therefore essential to maintain joint range and prevent severe contractures.

Management
Steroids may be successful.
Physiotherapy as for subacute dermatomyositis (see p. 164)

TALIPES CALCANEOVALGUS

Cause
Unknown.

Pathological changes
Opposite condition to TEV foot everted, dorsiflexed. Shortening anterior tibial.

Management
Responds rapidly to normal stretching.
1. Encourage parents to stretch tight structures
2. Active free movements
3. Strapping 6–8 weeks
4. Serial splinting, night splintage
5. Surgery

HAEMOPHILIA A AND CHRISTMAS DISEASE

Haemophilia A – a deficiency of Plasma Factor viii.
Christmas disease – a deficiency of Plasma Factor ix.
Both caused by sex-linked recessive genes.
Carried by females transmitted to males.
In early childhood prolonged bleeding follows minor trauma.
Weight-bearing joints most affected.

Management
1. Rest in acute phase (2 days) must be followed immediately with graded exercises to strengthen and mobilize
2. Hydrotherapy essential treatment
3. Prolonged splintage rarely used

OSTEOGENESIS IMPERFECTA (BRITTLE BONES)

Cause
Familial tendency (often Mediterranean type).

Pathological changes
A systemic disorder of mesenchyme (scleras, ligaments, bones). Defective osteoblastic activity.
Recurrent fractures occurring throughout life resulting in:
1. Skeletal deformities
2. Limb shortening
3. Gradual loss of independent ambulation
4. Deafness can occur in later life
5. Affected children may have blue sclera

Management
1. Improve function
    (i) Hydrotherapy
    (ii) Mobilize, strengthen regime
2. Guard against fractures
3. Maintain confidence (fear of trauma)
4. Prevention of deformities
    (i) Weight bearing when possible to prolong ambulation
    (ii) 'Moon suit' for walking

Some congenital limb abnormalities
1. Amelia – absence of a limb
2. Hemimelia – absence of portion of a limb
3. Phocomelia – reduction in size of proximal part of limb with approach of distal part towards trunk
4. Acheiria – absence of hand
5. Apodia – absence of foot
6. Polydactyly – supernumerary of fingers or toes
7. Syndactyly – fusion of bone, webbing of skin of hands or feet

Causes
1. Drugs in utero
2. Irradiation
3. Intra-uterine pressure
4. Genetic determination
5. Maternal age

Management
1. Encourage normal developmental sequence
2. Supervision of appropriate prosthesis and training
3. Support parents
4. Passive stretching (syndactyly)
5. Mobilize and strengthen (especially glutei)

JUVENILE RHEUMATOID ARTHRITIS (Still's disease)

See Diseases of joints page 149.

Physiotherapy management
1. Relieve pain
    (i) Analgesics
    (ii) Ice therapy
2. Prevent deformity
    (i) Short-term splintage during flare up
    (ii) Working splints to maintain wrist position
    (iii) Correct positioning in bed
    (iv) Encourage prone lying on bed with feet over ends of bed when resting
    (v) Advise suitable shoes, avoid high heels for teenagers
    (vi) Supervise any shoe adaptations i.e. insoles etc.
    (vii) Discourage slippers
3. Maintain mobility
    (i) Hydrotherapy daily
    (ii) Postural exercises
    (iii) Daily exercise regime – full active movements in all joints – do not forget neck, hands, fingers, toe joints
    (iv) Playing musical instrument
    (v) Daily walk
    (vi) Tricycle or bicycle essential (provide mobility when pain present)
    (vii) Encourage independent dressing etc.

14. Physiotherapy in mental handicap

Definition
The branch of physiotherapy dealing with the remedial and social aspects of the mentally handicapped.

MENTAL HANDICAP

A condition of 'mental impairment' or 'severe mental impairment' of such a degree that the person is incapable of living an independent life.

Causes
1. Genetic
2. Perinatal
3. Acquired
4. Unknown
1. Genetic
   (i) Chromosomal
       a. Down's syndrome
       b. Patau's syndrome
       c. Edwards' syndrome
       d. Cri-du chat syndrome
       e. Turner's syndrome
       f. Klinefelter's syndrome
       g. Triple X syndrome
       h. Tuberous sclerosis (epiloia)
       i. Apert's syndrome
       j. Ataxia telangiectasia (see p. 174).
   (ii) Possible genetic cause
       a. 'Happy puppet' syndrome
       b. De Lange syndrome
       c. Naevoid amentia (Sturge-Weber syndrome)
       d. Prader-Willi syndrome
   (iii) Metabolic
       a. Phenylketonuria
       b. Hyperglycaemia
       c. Maple syrup urine disease

      d. Lowe's syndrome
      e. Glycogen storage disorders
      f. Tay-Sachs' disease
      g. Batten's disease
      h. Leucodystrophy
      i. Gaucher's disease
      j. Hurler's syndrome
      k. Gargoylism
2. Perinatal
  (i) Trauma
  (ii) Anoxia
3. Acquired
  (i) Maternal infections
      a. Rubella
      b. Cytomegalovirus infection
      c. Varicella (chicken-pox)
      d. Syphilis
      e. Toxoplasmosis
  (ii) Childhood infections
      a. Encephalitis
      b. Meningitis
  (iii) Trauma
      a. Non-accidental injury
      b. Road traffic and home accidents
      c. Interruption of blood supply to brain e.g. cardiac arrest
      d. Irradiation
      e. Rhesus factor incompatibility
  (iv) Poisoning
      a. Lead, copper, manganese, strontium
      b. Carbon monoxide
  (v) Isolation amentia
4. Unknown
  A number (20–30%) of cases of mental handicap have no
  known cause

COMMON PROBLEMS ASSOCIATED WITH MENTAL HANDICAP

1. Microcephaly
2. Hydrocephaly (see p. 170)
3. Cerebral palsy (see p. 166)
4. Hemiplegia (see p. 167)
5. Spastic diplegia (see p. 166)
6. Visual impairment
7. Hearing impairment

The physiotherapist is involved with the physical problems related
to these, and other conditions where mental handicap is present.

Physical problems
1. Spasticity
2. Flaccidity
3. Deformities
4. Inco-ordination
6. Lack of balance
6. Deviant patterns of movement
7. Developmental milestones not achieved, or delayed

MANAGEMENT OF THE MENTALLY HANDICAPPED PERSON

Team approach.
All members assess on referral and discuss.

Team members
Physiotherapist
Occupational therapist
Speech therapist
Psychologist
Nurse/health visitor
Doctor
Social worker
Educational representative
The role of the physiotherapist is to maintain a watching brief, with episodes of intervention as required, throughout the life of the mentally handicapped person.

Assessment
1. To identify the problems, with diagnosis if possible, so that all team members and relatives, can understand the current situation
2. To predict what needs are likely to be
3. To provide a starting point for investigations and treatment
4. To review progress at subsequent intervals
The aim of multi-disciplinary intervention is to maximize the mentally handicapped person's potential, to enable him to be as independent as possible and to take his place in society.

Physiotherapists
1. Observe
2. Handle
3. Damp down unwanted postures, muscle tone and patterns of movement
4. Facilitate wanted postures, muscle tone and patterns of movement

Specific areas to be assessed and 'next steps' teaching programmes set up.

1. Gross motor
   - (i) Head control
   - (ii) Rolling
   - (iii) Sitting balance
   - (iv) Crawling
   - (v) Pull to standing
   - (vi) Side stepping
   - (vii) Walking
   - (viii) Running
   - (ix) Jumping
   - (x) Hopping
   - (xi) Pedalling
2. Fine motor
   - (i) Grasping, reaching
   - (ii) Clasp/unclasp hands
   - (iii) Transfer object from hand to hand
   - (iv) Pincer grasp
   - (v) Release object
   - (vi) Rolling object
   - (vii) Throwing object
   - (viii) Pointing, poking
   - (ix) Eye hand co-ordination
     - a. Stacking, building
     - b. Use of crayons
     - c. Threading beads, tying laces, fastening buttons etc.
3. Mental development
   - (i) Visual discrimination
   - (ii) Attention span
   - (iii) Permanence of objects
   - (iv) Exploration
   - (v) Relation of objects
   - (vi) Problem solving
   - (vii) Imitation
   - (viii) Discrimination
4. Personal – social
   - (i) Feeding
   - (ii) Communication, including speech
   - (iii) Emotional behaviour
   - (iv) Anticipation and expectation
   - (v) Play
   - (vi) Dressing
   - (vii) Toilet
   - (viii) Washing
   - (ix) Abstract concepts e.g. trust, loyalty, honesty
   - (x) Social interaction skills e.g. budgeting, road safety

Physiotherapy treatment
1. To maintain muscle tone in as normal a state as possible
    (i) Passive movements
    (ii) Patterning and positioning e.g. Bobath techniques
    (iii) Hydrotherapy
    (iv) Hot/cold therapies
        N.b. Drug therapy can influence muscle tone
2. To prevent deformities and maintain normal postures
    (i) Passive movements
    (ii) Active exercises
    (iii) Special mass produced equipment e.g. chairs, side lying boards
    (iv) Custom built equipment e.g. matrix chairs
    (v) Splintage
3. To prevent unwanted patterns of movement and facilitate normal patterns
    (i) Passive movements
    (ii) Active exercises
    (iii) Assisted exercises
        a. Slings
        b. Manual assistance
        c. Splints e.g. cock-up wrist splint with pencil incorporated
4. To enhance awareness of and interaction with surroundings
    (i) Tactile stimulation
        a. Texture boards; sandpaper, fur etc.
        b. Vibration therapy
        c. Rebound therapy
        d. Ball pool
        e. Soft play therapy
        f. Hydrotherapy
        g. Sand/water play
        h. Cuddling, touch play
        i. Different tastes and smells
        j. Horse-riding and other sports
    (ii) Auditory stimulation
        a. Music
        b. Speech
        c. General sounds – traffic, washing machine etc.
            Listening to and participating in groups and one-to-one situations
    (iii) Visual stimulation
        a. Flash cards, words and pictures
        b. Lights, torches; white and coloured
        c. 'Eye play' games, e.g. 'I Spy', 'Peek-a-Boo'
        d. Film, theatre, ballet etc.
    (iv) Social interaction
        a. Shops, cafes, restaurants, theatres
        b. Clubs

c. Sports activities
d. Holidays
e. Other people's houses

Early identification and intervention is essential if physical problems are to be minimized. Physiotherapy advice and/or treatment, in conjunction with other team members, should be available in a variety of settings:

1. The client's own home
2. Pre-school development assessment clinic
3. Pre-school parent/child groups
4. Health service provision
   (i) Day care: children/adults
   (ii) Residential care: children/adults
       a. Long term: children/adults
       b. Short term: children/adults
                     planned for treatment
                     planned for family relief
                     crisis
5. Special (and sometimes mainstream) education
6. Social services
   (i) Residential
       a. Hostels
       b. Group homes
       c. Substitute family care schemes
   (ii) Day care
       a. ATCs
       b. Day centres
       c. Luncheon clubs
       d. Sheltered workshops
7. Voluntary groups

FURTHER READING

Clarke, A. M. & Clarke, A. D. B. (eds) (1974) *Mental Deficiency – The Changing Outlook.* 3rd edition. London: Methuen.
Cunningham, C. & Sloper, P. (1978) *Handling your Handicapped Baby.* London: Souvenir Press.
Finnie, N. R. (1974) *Handling the Young Cerebral Palsied Child at Home.* 2nd edition. London: Heinemann Medical.
Heaton-Ward, W. A. (1976) *Mental Subnormality.* 4th edition. Bristol: Wright
Kirmen, B. & Bicknell, J. (1975) *Mental Handicap.* Edinburgh: Churchill Livingstone.
Portage Guide to Early Education. Portage Project CESA 12, Box 564, Portage, Wisconsin, 52901, USA.

15. The care and rehabilitation of the elderly

Introduction
This is a highly specialized field for physiotherapists. The elderly population is increasing in number and must no longer remain the 'poor relation' in health care. It necessitates an holistic approach to solve a variety of problems presented by the elderly and their carers.

The multi-pathology of many elderly people means that clinical aspects are only a small part of the overall picture.

Early intervention to prevent problems is essential, but physiotherapists must be aware that the remedial and social aspects are of equal importance.

Aims
The physiotherapist aims to:
1. *Prevent* deterioration in musculoskeletal system, balance and movement
2. *Motivate* the patient to achieve mutually agreed realistic goals – short-term and long-term
3. *Restore* and/or *maintain* optimum levels of independent movement and health (building confidence and giving encouragement)
4. Preserve the patient's *dignity*
5. Accurately *assess* and *review* patient's physical state, noting the individual's psychosocial and environmental needs
6. Work as part of the *multi-disciplinary team* (MDT)
7. *Share physiotherapy skills* as appropriate with others involved in caring for the elderly
8. *Evaluate* intervention and outcomes to check effectiveness

Multi-pathology
Multi-pathology is a major part of the problem facing many elderly people. Very rarely does a patient present with a single diagnosis, but several problems usually culminate to necessitate intervention. Here are listed some common problems for the elderly:

Alimentary disorders
1. Diarrhoea and vomiting
2. Hiatus hernia
3. Diverticulitis
4. Malabsorption
5. Carcinoma – oesophagus, stomach, colon, rectum
6. Constipation
7. Faecal incontinence from
    (i) Constipation – overflow incontinence
    (ii) Neurogenic
    (iii) Abuse of laxatives
    (iv) Symptomatic
        a. Side effects of drugs
        b. Diabetes
        c. Diverticular disease
        d. Carcinoma
        e. Rectal prolapse
        f. Poor mobility
8. Dysphagia

Anaemias
1. Iron deficiency
2. Megaloblastic
3. Of chronic disease
    (i) Chronic renal failure (uraemic)
    (ii) Rheumatoid
    (iii) Bowel disease
    (iv) Infected ulcers and pressure sores
    (v) Tuberculosis

Cardiovascular disorders
1. Myocardial infarction
2. Myocardial ischaemia (angina pectoris)
3. Intermittent claudication (angina cruris)
4. Gangrene – chronic leg ulcers
5. Hypertension
6. Postural hypotension
7. Heart valve disorders
8. Varicose veins
9. Varicose ulcers
10. Deep venous thrombosis
11. Congestive cardiac failure

Central nervous system disorders
1. CVA
    (i) Cerebral
    (ii) Cerebellar
    (iii) Brain stem

2. TIA
3. Cerebral atherosclerosis – see Dementia
4. Parkinsonism
5. Motor neurone disease
6. Multiple sclerosis
7. Other neurological disorders (see p. 55)

Diabetes
1. Mainly adult onset
2. Ulcers
3. Neuropathy

Dietary disorders (not as common as generally believed)
1. Scurvy (vitamin C deficiency)
2. Pellagra (vitamin B complex deficiency)
3. Vitamin B12 deficiency
4. Vitamin D deficiency.
5. Folate deficiency
6. Iron deficiency
7. Obesity – very common
8. Protein deficiency
9. Calcium deficiency

Ear disorders
1. Deterioration of hearing with age
2. Nerve deafness
3. Bone conduction deafness
4. Accumulation of wax
5. Ménière's disease
6. Ear infection

Eye disorders
1. Deterioration of vision
2. Glaucoma
3. Cataracts
4. Diabetic retinopathy
5. Hemianopea

Falls – possible causes
1. Cerebral
    (i) Drop attacks
    (ii) TIA
    (iii) Epilepsy
    (iv) 'Faints'
2. Cardiovascular
    (i) Postural hypotension
    (ii) Stokes-Adams attacks
3. Side effects of drugs

4. Failing eyesight
5. Lack of confidence
6. Environmental obstacles, e.g. furniture, stairs, scatter rugs
7. Decreased proprioception

Genitourinary disorders
1. Stress incontinence
2. Unstable bladder
3. Senile vaginitis
4. Chronic bacteriuria
5. Carcinoma of bladder
6. Prostatic hypertrophy
7. Neurogenic bladder
8. Urinary tract infection
9. Associated problems
    (i) Poor mobility
    (ii) Confusion or dementia
    (iii) Drugs e.g. diuretics

Homeostatic disorders
1. Electrolyte imbalance
    (i) Hypokalaemia (often from diuretics)
    (ii) Hyponatraemia
2. Dehydration
3. Hypothermia
4. Hyperthermia

Mental impairment
1. Dementia
    (i) Arteriosclerotic
    (ii) Alzheimer's disease
2. Confusion
    (i) Acute – due to infection, retention of urine, drugs etc.
    (ii) Long-standing – due to organic cerebral lesions, social changes, drugs etc.
3. Depression
    (i) Neurotic
    (ii) Psychotic

Musculoskeletal disorders
1. Osteoarthritis
2. Rheumatoid arthritis
3. Osteoporosis
4. Paget's disease
5. Osteomalacia
6. Tumours

Orthopaedic problems
1. Common fractures
    (i) Femoral neck – subcapital and transcervical
    (ii) Femoral – intertrochanteric and subtrochanteric
    (iii) Neck of humerus
    (iv) Colles'
    (v) Pubic ramus
    (vi) Head of radius
2. Joint replacement problems
3. Postoperative fixation problems
    (i) Protruding screws
    (ii) Loose pins

Pressure sores

Respiratory disorders
1. Bronchitis – acute and chronic
2. COAD
3. Pneumoconiosis
4. Pneumonias
5. Bronchiectasis
6. Asthma
7. Emphysema
8. Tuberculosis
9. Chest infections

Teeth
1. Poor fitting dentures
2. Bad teeth

Reasons for physiotherapy intervention
1. Inability to move independently
2. Poor mobility/history of falls
3. Chest problems
4. Social problems – patient and/or carer's fear of difficulty in coping
5. Pain
6. Apathy/depression/lack of confidence
7. Confusion
8. Altered muscle tone
9. Pressure sores
10. Incontinence

PRINCIPLES OF PHYSIOTHERAPY INTERVENTION

1. Assessment
   (i)   Patient's physical condition
   (ii) Patient's physiological condition
   (iii) Patient's social circumstances
   (iv) Patient's psychological state
2. Identify problems
3. Goal setting
   (i) Short-term aims
   (ii) Long-term aims
4. Total patient programme – mutually agreed between the patient (where possible), carers and physiotherapist
5. Monitoring – continual monitoring and re-assessment of the patient and his/her associated problems
6. *Evaluation*
   (i) Outcome of specific intervention
   (ii) Value of mutual experiences for future use

Team approach
Liaison between members of the team ensures all aspects of care will be covered – referral to other team members must be possible.

Team members
Hospital:

	Community:
Nursing staff	General practitioner
Physiotherapist	District nurse
Occupational therapist	Social services
Speech therapist	Community physiotherapist
Social worker	Health visitor
Doctors	Social worker
Dietician	Occupational therapist
Chiropodist	Chiropodist

While relatives/carers are not professional members of the MDT their part in the care and rehabilitation of the elderly is fundamental.

Ward rounds and conferences
Continual re-assessment and collation of information so that each team member is aware of progress and the aims and mode of treatment being given by each member. Communication is of paramount importance.

Encourage independence
The patient should contribute to his treatment by:
1. Dressing
2. Managing the toilet
3. Managing personal hygiene

4. Take own tablets
5. Walk whenever possible
6. Perform small tasks – butter bread etc.
7. Perform taught exercises on own
8. Talking to staff and other patients – important if speech problem

Discharge
Discuss with patient – assess attitudes
Discuss with involved relative – assess attitudes
Home visit essential if:
1. Patient residually disabled even if relative or help at home
2. Any change in environmental or social circumstances
Liaison with primary care team (community team).

Home visit
Take patient to home during the day with at least two team members – liaise with community team.

Aim
1. Assess ability to cope in own home
2. Decide if any equipment may be needed
3. Assess services required to support at home
Home visits can be done:
1. Early – reasons
    (i) Assess suitability of accommodation
    (ii) If major adaptations are necessary
    (iii) As morale booster or assess for weekend leave
2. Pre-discharge
    (i) Assess ability to cope
    (ii) Services required
    (iii) Assess for aids and adaptations
3. Discharge
    No problems anticipated: visit done on day of discharge as a final check

Resettlement in the community
Facilities available to support in the community (these may vary from area to area):
1. Warden service: daily check on the condition of the elderly person
2. District nurse: nursing care in the community
3. Home help: housekeeping tasks as assessed by home help supervisor
4. Meals on wheels or luncheon clubs
5. Community physiotherapist/occupational therapist: assessing, monitoring and intervention as necessary
6. Social services: referrals can be made to social services for

aids and adaptations in the home e.g. toilet aids, bath aids, ramps for wheelchair access, stairlifts
7. Social worker: becomes involved if problems develop outside the scope of the health team
8. Health visitor/geriatric visitor: makes visits to check patient is managing if district nurse is not involved
9. Laundry service
10. Bath attendants: under supervision of district nurse – normal bath or blanket bath
11. Twilight nurses/night attendants: help patients to bed or sit through the night if patients cannot manage themselves or relatives need relief
12. Chiropodist
13. Voluntary services: good neighbourhood schemes; 'Granny-sitting'

Other facilities to aid support in community
1. Day hospital
   Run by NHS with close attachment to a hospital. Reasons for attending:
   (i) Medical
   (ii) Physiotherapy
   (iii) Occupational therapy
   (iv) Speech therapy
   (v) Maintenance of severely disabled
   (vi) Social (for relative relief) when patient needs more care than available at day centres
2. Day centre: run by social services, sometimes allied to Part III home, to provide social stimulation, interaction and relative relief
3. Old age pensioner clubs: run by various charity groups, churches etc., e.g. Darby and Joan, over 60s
4. Luncheon clubs; health advisory clubs: run by health visitors
5. Voluntary transport schemes
6. ALAC
   Wheelchairs can usually be ordered from regional ALAC – self propelling or attendant chairs

Living accommodation available for the elderly
1. Their own home
2. With relatives/friends
3. Warden controlled accommodation
4. Sheltered housing
5. Housing associations
6. Part III accommodation run by social services
7. Private residential homes
8. Private nursing homes
9. Continual care hospital (NHS)

Case study
A 75-year-old obese diabetic woman with bronchopneumonia, mild
congestive cardiac failure and osteo-arthritic knees. Patient lives
alone in a small terraced house with outside WC and upstairs
bedroom; sole means of heating – coal fires. Her daughter
normally visits once per week. Until 4 weeks ago managed well
with help from a stick and neighbours who did a little shopping.
Fell in backyard 4 weeks ago. On ground for $\frac{1}{2}$ h. Found by
neighbour who helped her inside and called GP. No injury found,
but unable to get around due to pain and lack of confidence.
Therefore, sleeps on the settee and is at times incontinent due to
immobility. Daughter has stayed with mother since the fall, but this
has disrupted her own family life. 2 days ago developed cough and
pyrexia. Admitted to hospital.

Initial investigation
  1. Chest X-ray
  2. Check hips X-ray
  3. Urine analysis and culture
  4. Blood urea and electrolytes
  5. Full blood count
  6. Blood sugar
  7. Culture and sensitivity of sputum
  8. ECG

Treatment requested
  1. Broad spectrum antibiotic
  2. Mild diuretics
  3. Physiotherapy
  4. Diet for obesity and diabetes
  5. Analgesia for painful joints
  6. Monitor incontinence

Physiotherapy
Full assessment
Problems identified:
  1. Poor chest expansion and difficulty expectorating
  2. Painful stiff knees and slight flexion contracture of right knee
  3. Swollen ankles
  4. Fear or inability to move independently
  5. Incontinent
  6. Confusion (acute)
  7. Home environment will need adapting
  8. Strained relationship with daughter due to the disruption of
     daughter's family life

Goal setting – short term
Help alleviate chest problems and maintain clear chest, reduce

pain, increase muscle strength and range of movement. Teach exercise and care programme to help alleviate swollen ankles.

Goal setting – long term
Restore patient's confidence, independence and mobility. Assess home conditions – aids and adaptations. Discuss progress with daughter and assess attitudes.

Total patient programme
N.b. Although the acute confusion will resolve itself the physiotherapist must be aware that the patient will need reassurance and encouragement of this in the early stages.
1. Modified postural drainage (due to CCF)
   Breathing exercises
   Gentle percussion and vibration
   Encourage deep cough to remove secretions
2. Heat or ice to knees (constant attendance and checking of skin is necessary while patient still confused)
   Simple bed exercises with particular attention to knee and ankle joints

Progression
1. Encourage breathing exercises to maintain clear chest
2. Ensure legs are elevated as necessary and assess for support stockings and encourage exercises with feet elevated
3. Continue heat or ice and exercises progressing to standing and walking exercises, giving constant encouragement and help alleviate fear
   (i) On parallel bars
   (ii) With frame
   (iii) With stick
4. Check patient able to get in and out of bed and move around in bed
5. Practise climbing stairs and walking on uneven surfaces
6. Practise ability to get up off floor
7. Check with occupational therapist activities of daily living
   (i) Dressing
   (ii) Personal hygiene
   (iii) Kitchen
8. Discuss progress with patient and daughter
9. Regular reports at case conferences and ward rounds

Evaluation
Chest clear
Pain reduced
Walks independently with stick
Has overcome fear and lack of confidence in moving independently
Can climb stairs with stair rail

Cannot get up from floor unaided
Oedema of ankles controlled; can manage support stockings
Incontinence resolves when patient becomes independently mobile
Patient orientated in time and space

Plan for discharge
1. Patient very anxious to return home
2. Daughter happy to resume support as prior to the fall
3. Home visit planned – community team informed

Home visit
Members of team:
1. Physiotherapist
2. Occupational therapist
3. Social worker
4. Home help organizer
5. Daughter will meet the team at the home
To assess possible problems. Can she:
1. Manage stairs
2. Walk to outside toilet
3. Make up coal fire
4. Prepare meals in her own kitchen

Results
1. Second stair rail required as patient is anxious to sleep upstairs
2. Manage to get to outside toilet – but advise commode upstairs for night-time use
3. Difficulty lighting fire – home help organizer suggests fire lighting service – will arrange
4. Patient can prepare a simple meal and understands her diet
5. Daughter will do shopping and heavy washing once a week
6. Heavy cleaning to be done by home help once per week
Return to hospital and all services arranged.

On discharge
Day hospital – to maintain a check on her diabetes, dieting and mobility
Home help – once a week for cleaning and daily fire lighting service
Community physiotherapist – to check patient is managing at home

Guidelines for community psysiotherapy
1. As a member of the primary health care team (with hospital links) the physiotherapist may be based in the community at a health centre or have her base in the hospital. Some community physiotherapists have special responsibilities for Part III homes
2. Referrals may come from any other member of the primary

health care team or the hospital, but patients' GPs should be informed of the physiotherapist's intervention
3. Be aware of the variety of other back-up services to which patients can be referred e.g. day hospitals, day centres, good neighbour schemes
4. Written communication for relatives and other members of the primary health care team is essential
5. Always carry identification
6. The advisory and educational role of the physiotherapist to the patient and carers predominates
7. Be aware of the problems and stress carers endure and offer support
8. Remember if the patient is in his own home the physiotherapist is a guest and must adapt to the host's routine. Attitudes may differ from hospital environment
9. Social and environmental problems may broaden the range of physiotherapy intervention
10. Professional isolation exists, so ideally 3–4 years general physiotherapy experience is advisable before working in the community
11. Preventative and health education roles are important
12. Counselling skills are necessary to cope with bereavement, terminal care and family problems

FURTHER READING

Anderson, F. (1976) Preventative aspects of geriatric medicine. *Physiotherapy*, **62**, 5, 146.

Anderson, W. F. (1971) *Practical Management of the Elderly*. Oxford: Blackwell Scientific.

Anderson, W. F. & Judge, T. G. eds. (1974) *Geriatric Medicine*. London: Academic Press.

Brocklehurst, J. C. (1970) *The Geriatric Day Hospital*. London: King Edward's Hospital Fund.

Brocklehurst J. C. (1976) The day hospital. *Physiotherapy*, **62**, 5, 148.

Brocklehurst, J. C. & Hanley, T. (1976) *Geriatric Medicine for Students*. Edinburgh: Churchill Livingstone.

Caird, F. I. (1976) Diagnosis in old people. *Physiotherapy*, **62**, 6, 178.

Cash, J. E. (1985) *Neurology for Physiotherapists*. London: Faber & Faber.

Goble, J. E. & Nichols, P. J. R. (1971) *Rehabilitation of the Severely Disabled*. London: Butterworth.

Gray, M. & McKenzie, H. (1980) *Take Care of Your Elderly Relative*. London: Allen & Unwin.

Hawker, M. (1974) *Geriatrics for Physiotherapists and Allied Professions*. London: Faber & Faber.

Hinchcliffe, R. (1983) *Hearing and Balance in the Elderly*. Edinburgh: Churchill Livingstone

Hodkinson, H. H. (1981) *An Outline of Geriatrics*. London: Academic Press.

Isaacs, B. (1965) *Introduction to Geriatrics*. London: Baillere.

Isaacs, B. (1976) The place of a stroke unit in geriatric medicine, *Physiotherapy*, **62**, 5, 152.

Judge, T. G. (1976) Nutrition in the elderly, *Physiotherapy*, **62**, 6, 179.

Kennedy, B. F. (1976) The stroke unit: A physiotherapist's view, *Physiotherapy*, **62**, 5, 154.

Kennedy, R. D. (1976) Teamwork in geriatric medicine, *Physiotherapy*, **62**, 5, 158.

Mandelstam, D. A. (1976) Incontinence, *Physiotherapy*, **62**, 6, 182.

Mandelstam, D. A. (1980) *Incontinence and its Management*. London: Croom Helm.

Mary Marlborough Lodge eds. (1974) *Equipment for the Disabled*. 3rd edition. Nos 1–10. London: National Fund for Research into Crippling Diseases.

Marston, P. D. (1976) Day hospitals: A physiotherapist's view, *Physiotherapy*, **62**, 5, 151.

Robinson, R. A. (1976) Mental Illness in the elderly, *Physiotherapy*, **62**, 5, 155.

Index